W9-BNQ-868

Yoga Chick

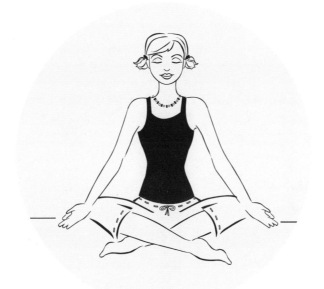

Yoga Chick

A Hip Guide to Everything Om

Bess Gallanis

Illustrations by Sheila MacDiarmid

WARNER BOOKS

NEW YORK   BOSTON

If you purchase this book without a cover, you should be aware that this book may have been stolen property and reported as "unsold and destroyed" to the publisher. In such case neither the author nor the publisher has received any payment for this "stripped book."

Neither this exercise program nor any other exercise program should be followed without first consulting a health care professional. If you have any special conditions requiring attention, you should consult with your health care professional regularly regarding possible modification of the program contained in this book.

Copyright © 2006 by Bess Gallanis, Inc.
All rights reserved.

Warner Books
Time Warner Book Group
1271 Avenue of the Americas, New York, NY 10020
Visit our Web site at www.twbookmark.com.

Printed in the United States of America

First Edition: January 2006
10 9 8 7 6 5 4 3 2 1

Library of Congress Cataloging-in-Publication Data

Gallanis, Bess.
Yoga chick: a hip guide to everything Om/Bess Gallanis—1st ed.
   p. cm.
ISBN 0-446-69432-0
1. Hatha yoga. 2. Women—Health and hygiene.
RA781.7.G353 2005
613.7'046—dc22

2005043815

Book design and text composition by JAM design
Cover design by Brigid Pearson

To Rick,

for helping me find my balance

in life's roughest waters

Acknowledgments

I gratefully acknowledge these treasured companions and fellow travelers on the long and exciting journey that was this book:

The journey simply would not have been possible had it not been for the OmGurl advisory board: Ava Friedman, Sarah Henschel, Talia Pines, Lily Seglin, Margaret Sharp, Nora Sharp, Samantha Sleeper and Paaven Thaker. These teenage yoginis inspired me to write about yoga in a way that was serious but not stuffy, fun but not frivolous. They were a source of imaginative ideas, courageously voiced their opinions, and were their truest selves. Their friendship is one of the many special gifts of this project. I thank each of them with all my heart.

My husband, Richard Hayes, lived and breathed this work with me, and it is enriched by his thoughtful contributions. Thank you, darling, for your loyal support, your love, and the many laughs we shared getting tangled up on my yoga mat.

To my wonderful agent, Laurie Abkemeier, thank you for your patient guidance, sensitive editorial touch, loyal support, and friendship. My lovely editor, Leila Porteous, added style and panache to this project, and I thank her for being my faithful advocate at Warner Books. No one could have wished for a more talented collaborator than Sheila MacDiarmid, who brought *Yoga Chick* to life through her illustrations.

Many people in the yoga world generously opened their hearts and studios and contributed ideas, feedback, friendship, and support. Ilene Sang and Marlene Mikel invited me into the calm world they created each Monday afternoon in their charming studio, Heart Center, in Highland Park, Illinois. Their expert insight as teachers, mothers, and friends is greatly appreciated.

Marsha Wenig, founder of YogaKids International, guided me through the process of writing about yoga in English. She kept me going with her warm and wise encouragement. Christy Brock, Leah Kalish, Holiday Johnson, and Dayna Macy contributed their expertise working with teenagers, and endless enthusiasm and support.

Thank you to Sharon Steffensen, publisher of *Yoga Chicago*. Her integrity and sound editorial judgment are gifts to her readers.

Lourdes Paredes and Christine Roy, partners in the lovely Namaskar yoga boutique and studio in Chicago, have been inspirational teachers and loving friends during this journey. They also kept me well dressed in stylish yoga clothes! Many thanks to my teachers and friends from Healing Power—Zoe Kaufman and Pam Udell—and Darren Friesen from Moksha. Blessings to Lane Jaabay and Amy Banasky of Innersy.

The unconditional love of my family has always been my sustenance: Mom, Stephanie, Connie and Lee, Peter and Chris, and Mom and Dad H., you make it possible for me to get up and take risks every day.

My Friday-morning friends at Marlene's Nail Emporium kept me well groomed and laughing.

Brenda Sexton and Dallas Jamison courageously led by example, and I thank them.

A big thanks to Wendy Goldman-Rohm. This work was conceived in her Master's Tea writers' workshop.

And to my tribe of wise women, my true source of strength, courage, and wisdom: Julie, Leslie, Maureen, Mary, Jenna, and Hannah. Thank you so very much, my friends.

Contents

Your Very Own Om

Yoga Chick: *A hip young yogini who embraces all life's possibilities on and off her yoga mat.*

I have practiced yoga for many years, but my work on this book began when I met Ava Friedman, a passionate yogini who found inspiration in the natural yoga lifestyle on and off her mat.

Yoga was a welcome break at the end of Ava's busy day and helped her to relax. "Yoga makes me feel so good," she told me over a steaming cup of latte after class one snowy, cold Saturday afternoon. "And you can really work up a sweat and build muscles." Ava also enjoyed activities that enhanced her yoga experience, like exploring her thoughts through journaling, learning about the chakras, and trying to meditate.

Ava had discovered the yoga lifestyle and its balance between body, mind, and emotions as the foundation for lifelong wellness. And she is not alone. Over the next several months, I reached out to young women like Ava to learn more about how they viewed yoga and its role in their busy lives. Over gallons of green tea smoothies and chai lattes, young women talked about their bodies and health, their lives and passions.

Yoga Chicks practice to work up a sweat, build muscles, and increase their strength, stamina, and flexibility. But yoga isn't just about how you look, it is also about how you feel. Yoga asks you to slow down, look inward, clear the chatter from your mind, and develop a relationship with an important person in your life: yourself.

Yoga Chick: A Hip Guide to Everything Om has pulled together all the tools you will need to lead a healthy, natural yoga lifestyle:

@ Six complete yoga practices that fit your busy schedule

@ Breathing exercises that get you fired up

@ Relaxation techniques to calm you down

@ Self-reflection exercises

@ Self-care to enhance your well-being

@ Delicious recipes for healthy eating

The book is organized to reflect a typical day in the life of a Yoga Chick. Each chapter stands on its own and includes an efficient and effective yoga practice, discussion of an authentic yoga principle, a self-reflection exercise, self-care and nutrition tips—and more.

Let the practice inspire you!

Peace,
Bess Gallanis

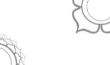

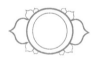

PART I

Yoga Chick

101

CHAPTER ONE

Yoga's Ancient Beginnings

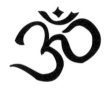

Yoga originated in India more than five thousand years ago. Inspired by Hindu mythology and later influenced by Buddhism, it is an ancient lifestyle that promotes natural approaches to health and wellness. Though many people seek spirituality through their yoga practice, it is not a religion in the traditional sense. Yoga is the philosophy of uniting the mind, body, and spirit: One who is at peace with herself is in harmony with other people, nature, and the universe.

Nearly two thousand years ago, an Indian philosopher named Patanjali defined yoga in a book called the *Yoga Sutra*. Patanjali condensed thousands of years of yoga tradition into 195 brief passages that defined the health practices, breathing exercises, meditation practices, and moral code of the yoga lifestyle.

After *Yoga Sutra* was published, yoga continued to evolve. Sri T. Krishnamacharya, an influential Indian teacher and healer who lived during the twentieth century, taught people how to coordinate their breath while performing a continuous series of poses to create the active yoga practice called Flow yoga.

Building on his work, three of Krishnamacharya's students developed their own yoga styles that define contemporary yoga practices. Pattabhi Jois developed Ashtanga yoga, also known as power yoga. B. K. S. Iyengar developed the Iyengar style of yoga, which is also referred to as gentle yoga. He taught people to adapt yoga poses to their physical ability by using props like blocks, straps, chairs, and bolsters. T. K. V. Desikachar introduced Viniyoga, which promotes yoga practice as a vehicle for self-discovery and personal growth.

The *Yoga Sutra* summarizes the main principles of the yoga lifestyle in the Eight-Limbed Path. The Eights Limbs are moral discipline, self-reflection, exercise and healthy habits, controlling the breath, looking inward without becoming distracted, sustained concentration, meditation, and finding ultimate peace.

It would take a lifetime of study and devotion to each of the Eight Limbs to have a full appreciation for what it takes to travel the yoga path to finding ultimate peace. In *Yoga Chick* we practice the basics: yoga poses, breathing techniques, and meditation. Once you get the hang of these fundamental skills, you will be well on your way to a healthy and natural lifestyle.

CHAPTER TWO

Going With the Yoga Flow

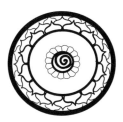

In the last hundred years, yoga has evolved to fit the needs of people in the West. Yoga is based on five-thousand-year-old principles that guide each and every practice even today. These principles are incorporated into each chapter to help you get the most benefit from your yoga practice.

Yoga Chick is based on the yoga-flow philosophy. Each yoga practice is like a dance: a continuous sequence of poses that are coordinated by inhaling and exhaling your breath. Flow challenges you to coordinate your body, your breathing, and your attitude as you progress from one pose to the next.

The yoga-flow philosophy also reflects the natural cycles of nature. It is a creative way to develop sensitivity to your natural energy patterns. When you listen to your body, it will tell you what it needs: rest, exercise, food, or pampering. Flow cultivates your intuition so that you become perceptive about your behavior and habits. Each chapter in this book offers new ideas that will help you manage your physical energy, tune in to your feelings, let go of distracting thoughts, find mental balance, and deal with change.

Three-Part Harmony: The Mind-Body-Spirit Connection

The mind, body, and spirit are deeply connected through yoga. Breathing exercises help you manage your physical energy and develop concentration. Regular yoga practice supports good health and develops self-discipline. Meditation cultivates a calm, peaceful attitude and self-awareness. When your mind, body, and spirit are balanced, you are completely in tune with yourself. You have reached a state of "flow."

Yoga Practice, Not Yoga Perfect

Yoga gives you the chance to practice without the pressure of performance. Some days you will perform challenging yoga poses with grace and confidence. Other days you will struggle to move into the very same pose. Do not expect to master yoga poses every time you step on your mat. Yoga is about how you feel in a pose, not how you look. Whether you are a beginner or an experienced yoga student, no one ever masters yoga, because there is always something more we can learn about ourselves. Every yoga practice is an exercise in self-exploration. This is why it is called practice.

Standing on Your Own Two Feet

Each yoga practice begins by making a firm connection to the earth. This is called "getting grounded." You are grounded when you are standing firmly and calmly, aware of your feet touching the floor and attentive to your surroundings.

STANDING STILL LEADS TO INNER PEACE

A yoga pose has two layers of meaning: physical and philosophical. We practice yoga to develop flexibility, strength, balance, and resilience in our bodies and our minds.

Yoga poses that improve flexibility rely on stretching to increase the body's range of motion. With a little stretching, your muscles will release and open farther than you ever thought possible. The same is true in your life. A person who is willing to be mentally flexible is open-minded to new ideas rather than fixed or rigid in their thinking. You never know what will happen until you are open to new possibilities.

Poses that increase strength and endurance demand focus, concentration, and commitment to stick with it even when the going gets tough. Achieving our goals in life require us to focus and commit for long periods of time, sometimes for years.

Balance poses can be powerful and dynamic, demanding both strength and flexibility, effort and release, focus and joy. Creating balance in our lives is a dynamic process, too. Often we must weigh competing priorities, like family and friends, study and work. Yoga practice can provide a different way to look at things in your life so that you can make good decisions that serve your best interests.

Try this: Stand in Mountain Pose (page 13). Get grounded and pay attention to your alignment. Feel all four corners of each foot pressing into the floor. Flex your toes and raise them from the floor. When you feel balanced and strong, open your eyes and smile. You just learned how to stand on your own two feet.

Wide Awake

Yoga asks you to wake up to reality by staying alert and paying attention during practice. Only then can you be open to new physical sensations in your body and the thoughts that cross your mind. By observing how you react to situations—challenge and success, frustration and joy—you develop self-awareness. So much of our behavior is nothing more than habit. When you are aware of your own behavior, you can make wise and thoughtful choices—on your yoga mat and in your life.

Yoga Is an Action Verb

Yoga is often misunderstood to be a passive activity, but it is really about taking action. Every time you step onto your yoga mat, you are acting to improve your health and to know yourself. Sometimes you will summon the courage to push beyond your comfort zone in an effort to test and challenge yourself. Other days you will hang back, listening to your body and its plea for relaxation. Growth happens one pose at a time.

Sweet Surrender

In order to fully concentrate on your yoga practice, relax, and prepare for meditation, you will learn to calm your mind and let go of attachments. We become attached to our thoughts, our habits, our emotions, and our ways of thinking, even if they cause us pain. Concentrating on your breathing is the technique for learning how to let go of the thoughts that can distract you during your yoga practice. As you become more comfortable with letting go of your thoughts, you can begin to practice letting go of distracting emotions, such as anger or frustration.

Balancing Act

A fundamental principle of yoga is the concept of balance. Every yoga pose is a balancing act between strength and flexibility, exertion and relaxation, front and back. When you are out of balance, another part of your body bears the extra burden, creating aches and pains. What you learn on the mat about balance applies to life as well. Hard work must be counterbalanced by relaxation.

The Only Constant Is Change

Change is inevitable and everyone has to learn how to cope with changes in life. Some changes are expected and welcome. The seasons change in tune with nature, and we welcome spring's flowers and the butterflies of summer. Changes that happen too fast and take us by surprise knock us off balance. Changes imposed on us make us feel as if we have no control over our lives. It can be hard to keep your balance when you feel you have no control over the changes sweeping over your life. Yoga helps you to accept change by teaching you perspective and how to make smooth transitions.

EVERY BREATH YOU TAKE

You take between 20,000 and 30,000 breaths per day! In cultures that practice yoga, the breath is the tool they use to access their body's life force or spirit. In this book we simply refer to it as using the breath to access our energy—both physical and emotional.

Consciously controlled breathing is the foundation of yoga. Most stress management techniques focus on breath control—for good reason. Drawing a full breath increases the amount of oxygen that circulates through your body and into your brain and calms the sympathetic nervous system.

Yoga breathing helps us reach deep inside to the core of our bodies where we store our emotions. The ability to access our emotions and control our response to them is one of yoga's most valuable life lessons.

Authentic yoga breathing is controlled four ways: inhaling, exhaling, retaining your breath after inhaling, and retaining your breath after exhaling. *Yoga Chick* emphasizes inhaling and exhaling in its yoga practices.

Slowly inhale through your nose, breathing into your diaphragm, which is located beneath the V-shaped area below your rib cage. Exhale through your nose. Couldn't be simpler, but it might take some practice.

CHAPTER THREE

Getting Started

Before you begin any new physical fitness activity, check with your doctor, especially if you have been sick, suffer from a chronic illness, or have been injured. Most healthy young women should be able to perform the yoga poses in this book safely.

Starting Out on the Right Foot

Start with the Right Attitude

Yoga is not a competitive sport. It is an individual practice that changes every day depending upon your mood and energy level. Set your own goals and yoga will satisfy your needs. There is no failure in yoga.

Setting Up Your Home Studio

You can practice yoga just about anywhere. Choose a warm room with good energy and good light. You will need enough room to stretch your arms out in all directions. A mirror is not necessary and can be a distraction.

Keep It Simple

A yoga mat is nice, but not necessary. Yoga mats are made from rubber that has been coated with a sticky substance to prevent you from slipping during practice. You can also find mats that are extra thick to provide cushioning, or that are decorated with colorful graphics that can help with your alignment in a pose. A big beach towel can serve the same purpose as a yoga mat. Square foam blocks and D-ring straps are helpful props, too, especially when you are beginning a new yoga practice.

Create the Mood

Lightly scented incense or a scented candle creates a nice atmosphere. Just make sure you have enough ventilation in your practice area. Music can enhance yoga practice, too.

Warm Up

You will be more comfortable and avoid injury if you practice yoga when you are nicely warmed up. If you live in a cool climate, be sure to practice yoga in a warm room. A quick shower or bath will help you warm up, too.

Go with the Flow

Many of the practices in this book are yoga-flow sequences. Your breathing is synchronized with the movement of each yoga pose. In general, you reach up or out as you inhale and release or bend forward as you exhale. As you inhale, visualize your breath inflating your body like a balloon and expanding your joints. As you exhale, visualize your body contracting to squeeze out stress, negative feelings, and health-damaging toxins.

Practice Tips for Your Safety and Comfort

Each practice in this book is built upon a sequence of individual yoga poses. The sequence of poses has been carefully chosen so that you will get an effective, efficient, and balanced yoga practice. Read and review each pose, then practice once or twice in front of a mirror to create a visual memory of yourself.

Practice at Your Own Pace

As with any other physical activity, if you practice yoga incorrectly you can hurt yourself. If you practice regularly, your flexibility, strength, and concentration will improve. Move slowly and concentrate in each pose.

Listen to Your Body

Yoga should not hurt. Each pose offers you a chance for self-exploration. Listen to your body, and let it tell you how far to stretch or how long to hold a pose.

Visualize Yourself in a Pose

Bring the power of your imagination to your practice. Imagine your body taking shape in the pose, your joints opening as you stretch, and your limbs extending from your torso. Many yoga poses reflect animals and other elements from nature. Imagine yourself as a delicate swan or a silver half-moon and you will feel graceful and light.

Increase the Challenge Breath by Breath

When starting out, hold each yoga pose for three to five breaths. On the days you feel like a challenge, hold your poses longer. It's easy to vary the intensity of your practice from pose to pose by adjusting how long you stay in each one.

Wear Comfortable Clothes

You may want to treat yourself to a yoga outfit to inspire your practice, but you do not need special clothes. Wear comfortable clothes you would wear for exercise. Tights, loose-fitting pants, or shorts work well for yoga poses. It's a good idea to wear one or two layers on top, especially during the winter. Yoga is most effective, safe, and enjoyable when you are a little warm. You can always remove the second layer as you generate more body heat. Yoga is always practiced in bare feet, though you may want to have a pair of warm socks and a blanket handy to stay warm during a resting pose.

Practice on an Empty Stomach

To get the most from yoga, practice on an empty—or almost empty—stomach. You are safe drinking water, a small glass of juice or milk, or a cup of herbal tea. The rule of thumb is to practice yoga three hours after your last meal. You may safely eat a meal thirty minutes after practice.

Drink Lots of Fluids

After your practice, replenish your body's fluids by drinking plenty of water, a citrus spritzer, a cup of herbal tea, or a glass of milk. Even if you did not feel perspiration during practice, your body's fluids have evaporated through breathing.

MOUNTAIN POSE

Stand tall with your feet hip-width apart. Roll your shoulders back, arms at your sides with the palms facing your body and fingers pointed to the floor. To get grounded, distribute your weight evenly over both feet. Feel all four corners of your feet on the ground. Raise and lower your toes a few times to check your stability. Tuck your tailbone under, contract your abdomen, and extend your head from your neck for a nice, long spine. Look straight ahead or gaze down your nose. Visualize yourself as a strong and stable mountain and begin to focus on your breathing.

Mountain is the foundation posture for all standing yoga poses. It focuses your attention on standing on your own two feet.

STANDING ARM RAISE

Inhale: Raise your arms out to the sides of your body and reach up over your head. Reach toward the ceiling, feeling your spine lengthen.

Exhale: Lower your arms.

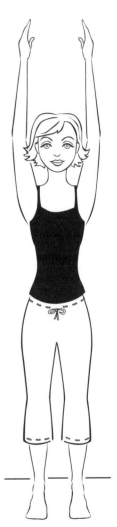

STANDING ARM RAISE WITH A BACK BEND

Inhale: Reach out from your shoulders, raise your arms out to the sides of your body, and reach up over your head, fingertips touching. Raise your chin to look up at your hands and continue to reach toward the ceiling, feeling your spine lengthen. When you feel stable and comfortable, bend back from the waist.

Exhale: Lower your arms to your sides and straighten your head and back.

As you become more flexible, work toward deepening your back bend. Visualize the crown of your head leading your back farther.

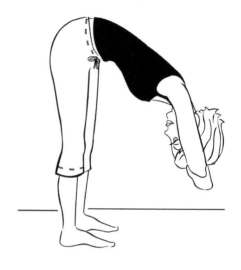

STANDING FORWARD FOLD, ARMS FOLDED

Inhale: Raise your arms out to the sides of your body and reach up over your head. Raise your chin to look up at your hands and continue to reach toward the ceiling, feeling your spine lengthen.

Exhale: Tuck your chin to your chest, bend forward from your waist, arms out to the side, palms facing down. Fold your arms one over the other, clasping your elbows. Bend your knees and point the crown of your head to the floor. Feel your lower back stretch. Stay in this position for a few breaths.

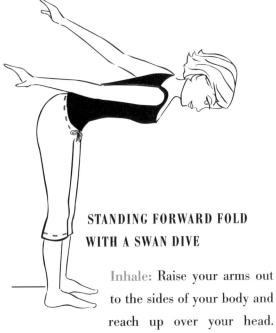

STANDING FORWARD FOLD WITH A SWAN DIVE

Inhale: Raise your arms out to the sides of your body and reach up over your head. Raise your chin to look up at your hands and continue to reach toward the ceiling, feeling your spine lengthen.

Exhale: Gracefully float your arms out to the side, palms facing down, bending forward from the waist. Touch the floor with your fingertips in front of your feet, bending your knees if necessary. If you are flexible enough, straighten your knees. Work toward pressing the entire palm of your hand to the floor and straightening your legs.

Linked by the rhythm of your breathing, arm raises and forward folds work together to create flow in your yoga practice. Adding a Swan Dive to your forward fold develops grace and flexibility. Start forward folds with your knees bent and work toward straightening your legs.

DOWN DOG

Start with your hands and knees on the floor or mat, arms shoulder-width apart and extended in front of you, palms pressed into the floor. Do not lock your elbows.

Inhale: Standing on the balls of your feet, lift your hips toward the ceiling and straighten your arms and legs. Tuck your chin and look back toward your belly button.

Exhale: Lower your heels to the ground. Continue to push your palms into the floor for stability, but let your legs do most of the work of holding you up. Continue pressing both heels to the floor.

Variations

- For a deeper stretch in the hamstrings, deeply bend one knee, then the other knee.
- To get a stretch through your hip flexor, bend a leg at the knee and squeeze it to your chest. Rotate your leg out to the side. You will be in the same position as a dog answering Mother Nature's call.
- For a little abdominal strengthening, inhale and raise your leg straight back and up to a comfortable height. Exhale and lower your leg, bent at the knee. Squeeze your knee into your chest and tuck your chin under.

Down Dog is a transition pose. You can take a break and hang out for a few breaths or move between standing and seated postures. Down Dog stretches the hamstrings and calves and builds strong arms.

DOG AND CAT POSE

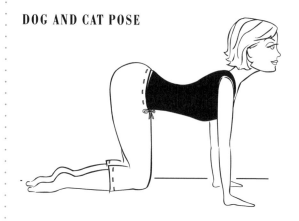

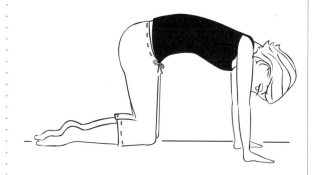

Starting from all fours, place your hands firmly on the floor directly below your shoulders, arms straight.

Inhale: Lift your chin, bending your head back—stretching your neck—and lift your tailbone, lowering your back as deeply as you can.

Exhale: Carefully tuck your chin to your chest—gently stretching your neck in the opposite direction—contract your abdominal muscles, and arch your back up. Use your breath to create a comfortable rhythm to loosen your spine from your neck all the way to your lower back.

Practiced regularly, the Dog and Cat Pose develops a flexible spine and tones the abs. Breathe deeply to inflate your backside for a deeper stretch.

CHILD'S POSE

Kneel on the floor with your feet together and your knees wide apart. Sit back on your heels. Bend forward from your waist over your knees. Place your forehead on the floor. Relax your shoulders and let your arms fall comfortably to the floor at your sides.

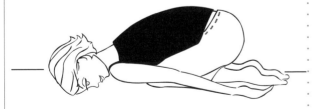

EXTENDED CHILD'S POSE

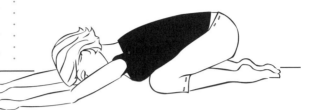

Kneel on the floor with your feet together and your knees wide apart. Sit back on your heels. Bend forward from your waist over your knees. Place your forehead on the floor. Try to lower your buttocks to your heels. Extend your arms straight out in front of you, palms flat on the floor.

Any time you need a break, melt into Child's Pose.

PEACEFUL POSE

Cooling down in meditative Peaceful Pose is an important part of yoga practice. It gives your body a chance to absorb the energy it produced during your yoga practice, energy that will continue to make you feel terrific long after you leave your mat. Use the time you lie in Peaceful Pose to relax, but remain alert and aware of how your body responds to this release. If your lower

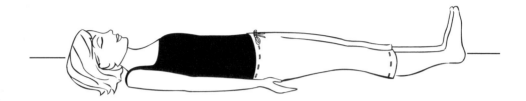

back is uncomfortable lying flat on the floor, prop up your knees with a blanket or bolster. It also is nice to use a scented eye pillow. Cover yourself with a blanket to stay warm.

Lie flat on your back on the floor with your arms and legs open a comfortable distance apart, but no more than a few inches. Breathe naturally.

Beginning with your feet, let go, totally relaxing. Feel the heels of your feet sink into the floor. Move up your body, consciously letting go at each point where your body touches the floor. Try not to think, just enjoy the feeling of sinking into the floor. Stay in this position as long as you like—but don't fall asleep!

PART II

Everyday Om

CHAPTER FOUR

Start the Day Off Right

*A little yoga first thing in the morning
makes you feel terrific all day!*

What kind of a morning person are you? Do you bound from bed with a smile on your face? Lucky you! Most of us hit the snooze button on the alarm, roll over, and cover our heads with a pillow. A little yoga in the morning helps you get grounded by making a firm connection to yourself and to your surroundings. Getting centered first thing in the morning creates a sense of well-being that lasts the whole day.

This yoga practice uses those early-morning deep yawns and cat stretches to ease you out of bed. Stretching is key to creating the long, supple muscles that support graceful movement. A round of full yoga breaths will warm and energize you and make your face glow, too.

This morning practice ends in Mountain, the foundation for all standing poses in yoga. But there is a lot more to it than standing around. It is a head-to-toe body survey that helps you develop self-awareness. It also improves your posture and balance. Stand tall with your feet pressing firmly into the floor, your head extending up from your neck and spine, and focus your mind's eye inward. Concentrate on your breath and begin to gather the self-confidence you will need to see you through the busy day ahead.

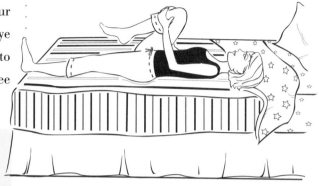

Practice tip: Morning practice is about learning to stand on your own two feet. To get the most from it, breathe deeply, stretch slowly, and stand confidently.

LYING ARM RAISE

Inhale: While still lying in bed, raise your arms over your head. Stretch your legs and flex your feet.

Exhale: Raise your arms straight up in the air and then lower them to your sides.

KNEE TO CHEST

Inhale: Bend your right leg at the knee. Holding your shin just below the knee, gently hug your leg to your chest.

Exhale: Lower your knee, extending your leg and flexing your foot.

Repeat with your left leg.

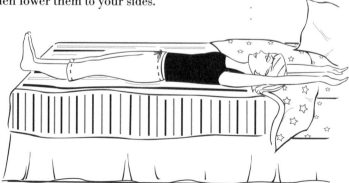

TWO KNEES TO CHEST

Inhale: Bend both legs at the knee. Hold your shins just below the knees and gently hug your legs to your chest.

Exhale: Lower your knees, extending your legs and flexing your feet.

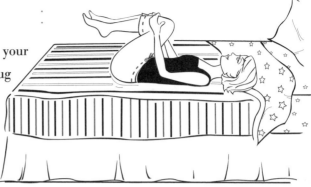

BREATHE DEEPLY: BASIC YOGA BREATHING TECHNIQUE

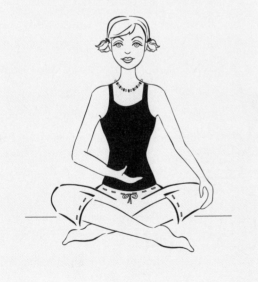

All of the yoga breathing exercises in this book are based on the classic three-part yoga breathing technique:

1. Take deep, controlled breaths through your nose.
2. Draw the breath into your diaphragm until it expands.
3. Use your abdominal muscles to control your exhalation.

To get the hang of it, stand in Mountain Pose and practice taking a few breaths through your nose. Take a deeper breath while you slowly count to three. Now, place your hand over your diaphragm, which is located beneath the

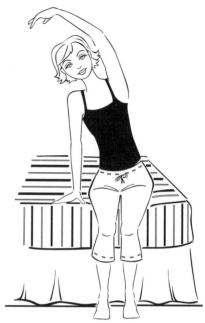

V-shaped area below your rib cage. Inhale into that spot and feel your abdomen rise as your diaphragm expands. Contract your abdomen and exhale through your nose.

To take a full yoga breath, inhale deeply, expanding your diaphragm and abdomen, letting your breath rise to fill your chest.

Yoga breathing may seem a little awkward at first, and you may feel a little lightheaded. With practice, yoga breathing will come naturally to you. You can practice your yoga breathing any-where and anytime.

SEATED HALF MOON

Inhale: Place your right hand, palm down, firmly on the bed at your side. Extend your left arm out to the side, palm up. Lift your left arm until it is straight overhead. Gently stretch your torso to the right as your left hand continues to reach up and over your head following your torso.

SEATED ARM RAISE

Inhale: Raise your arms out to the sides, palms facing up. Lift them above your head until your fingertips touch.

Exhale: Lower your arms to your sides.

Exhale: Straighten your torso and slowly lower your left arm to your side.

Repeat on the other side.

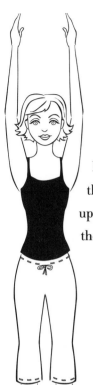

STANDING ARM RAISE

Inhale: Raise your arms out to the sides of your body and reach up over your head. Reach toward the ceiling, lengthening your spine.

STIMULATE YOUR SENSES

Some scents make us swoon because our sense of smell is connected directly to the brain and creates an instant and powerful emotional response.

Aromatherapy is the ancient practice of stimulating our scent receptors with the essential oils of flowers and herbs to calm us down or energize us. The right combination of scents first thing in the morning can naturally stimulate a happy mood and mental alertness, while a soothing fragrance in the evening can help us wind down from a busy, stressful day.

Many modern bath products are scented using the principles of aromatherapy. Rosemary and peppermint are invigorating and stimulating. Rosemary warms you up and improves concentration, while peppermint will cool you down and wake up your senses. Lemongrass is refreshing and promotes a happy frame of mind. Look for any of these scents, either alone or in combination, in shower gels and soaps.

If you are crafty, make your own morning shower gel by adding a few drops of your favorite essential oil to unscented liquid soap. For more tips, see "Fine-Tune Your Moods with Aromatherapy" on pages 95–96.

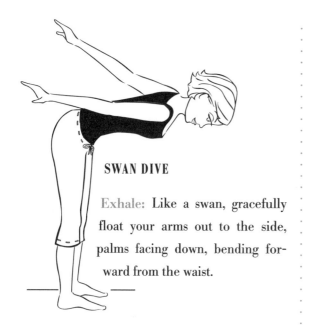

SWAN DIVE

Exhale: Like a swan, gracefully float your arms out to the side, palms facing down, bending forward from the waist.

STANDING FORWARD FOLD, ARMS FOLDED

Inhale: Tuck your chin to your chest, bend forward from your waist, arms out to the side, palms facing down. Fold your arms one over the other, clasping your elbows. Bend your knees and point the crown of your head to the floor. Feel your lower back stretch. Stay in this position for a few breaths.

DOG AND CAT POSE

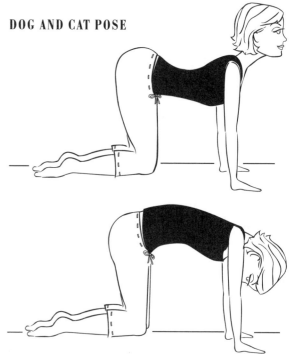

Starting on all fours, place your hands firmly on the floor directly below your shoulders, arms straight.

Inhale: Lift your chin and chest, bend your head back, lift your tailbone, and lower your back as deeply as you can.

Exhale: Carefully tuck your chin to your chest, contract your abdominal muscles, and round your back.

Repeat this sequence several times, using your breath to create a comfortable rhythm.

Breakfast really is the most important meal of the day. We think it's our bodies that need fuel, but really, it's our brains that need breakfast. Your brain is a ravenous beast and consumes about one-third of your daily calories just in the morning. To make the most of your breakfast calories you need protein, fiber, complex carbohydrates, and a little fat. The protein content in this smoothie will power up your brain and keep your appetite at bay until lunch. Supplement your smoothie with two pieces of buttered whole-grain toast or a bagel for a totally nutritious breakfast.

POWER SMOOTHIE

Choose ¾ cup from the following: whole, skim, 2%, soy, nut, or rice milk

Choose ¼ cup from the following: plain or vanilla-flavored yogurt, firm tofu

Choose ½ cup from the following: frozen or fresh strawberries, blueberries, cherries, mango, papaya, bananas

1 tablespoon Splenda, honey, stevia, or other natural sweetener

½ teaspoon vanilla extract

Combine all ingredients in a blender, mix to desired consistency, and enjoy!

Makes 1 serving

Yoga Chick Tips

- Facing a grueling morning? Supercharge your brain by boosting the protein content of your smoothie with a tablespoon of whey or soy powder.

- To gain a little extra energy, stoke your body's engine by adding half a banana and one tablespoon of creamy peanut butter.

- Feeling under the weather? Arm your immune system by adding one teaspoon of vitamin C powder.

If you're short on time in the morning, prepare your smoothie before going to bed and do the following:

- Store it in a resealable container and refrigerate. In the morning, reblend the smoothie with an ice cube and enjoy it while getting ready for, or on your way to, school.

- Freeze overnight in the same container you will drink it from. On your way out the door in the morning, grab the frozen smoothie and stow it in your backpack. By midmorning it should have thawed enough to drink. Shake vigorously and enjoy between classes.

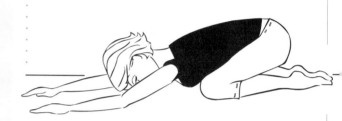

EXTENDED CHILD'S POSE

Start on all fours with knees shoulder-width apart and feet touching. Fold at the waist and knees, sitting on your calves and resting your chest on your knees, forehead touching the floor. Try to lower your bottom to your heels. Extend your arms straight out in front of you, palms flat on the floor. Stay here for a few breaths.

ABDOMINAL CRUNCHES

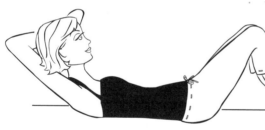

Inhale: Contract your abdomen, plant your lower back firmly on the floor, and lift your head and shoulders up from the floor.

Exhale: Slowly roll back down.

Repeat five to ten times.

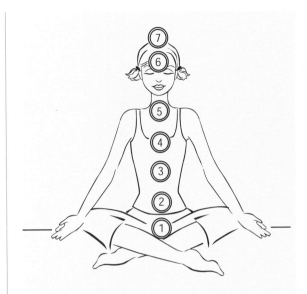

SPIN YOUR ENERGY WHEELS: THE CHAKRA SYSTEM

The chakras are spiraling wheels of energy that line up from the base of the spine to the top of the head. *Chakra* means "wheel of light" and each one represents a state of consciousness, beginning with our most primitive needs for security to our spiritual needs for peace of mind. You cannot touch the chakras, because they are not organs or nerves, but you can feel their impact on your health and emotions. When your body, mind, and spirit are in harmony and are working together cooperatively, chakra energy flows freely and drives creativity, discovery, journeys, relationships, integrity, and good health. You can stimulate your chakras through color choices, music, meditation, yoga practice, and affirmations. The affirmations are most powerful when spoken out loud at the beginning or after your yoga session or after meditation.

The Chakras

Root Chakra: Instinct

The first chakra is located at the base of the spine and repre-sents our most primitive nature and survival 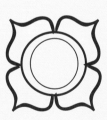 instincts. Because it influences our sense of security, a strong root chakra helps us stay grounded. To stimulate this chakra, wear the color red and practice Mountain Pose.

Affirmation: I am strong and secure and adapt to changes in my life by going with the flow.

Sacral Chakra: Creativity

The second chakra is located just below the navel and represents procreation and sexuality. Because it influences our most creative impulses, a  strong sacral chakra contributes to an overall sense of well-being. Indulge your inner child, take pleasure in the wonders of the world, and wear the color orange to stimulate this chakra.

Affirmation: I allow abundance and pleasure into my life.

Solar Plexus Chakra: Power

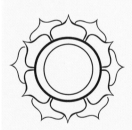 The third chakra represents personal power. It is the source of our identity, and the integrity that comes from learning to be your truest self. It begins to develop during high school. Vigorous exercise, especially abdominal work, and the color yellow stimulate this chakra.

Affirmation: I am confident in my growing intelligence and wisdom.

Heart Chakra: Compassion

The fourth chakra is the center of love and influences the development of our compassion for ourselves and others. Self-love is the most important  love of all. Practice breathing exercises and wear the color green to stimulate this chakra.

Affirmation: I love myself unconditionally.

Throat Chakra: Truth

The fifth chakra represents verbal expression and communication. It influences the expression of emotions and creates understanding. 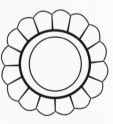 Bright blues, such as turquoise and aquamarine, express the clear communication and thinking that is the essential nature of this chakra. Writing and storytelling stimulate this chakra.

Affirmation: I express myself honestly and with integrity and believe the world is listening to me.

Brow Chakra: Wisdom

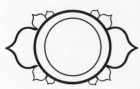

The sixth chakra is located in the forehead, the site of the Third Eye, and represents the intersection of our human instincts and intellect. It influences our imagination, intuition, and insight through self-reflection. Create visual art through drawing, painting, photography, or filmmaking, and wear the color purple to stimulate this chakra.

Affirmation: I see things clearly and can express my vision and imagination.

Crown Chakra: Peace

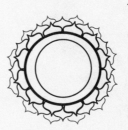

The seventh chakra governs higher consciousness. Enlightenment is peace of mind. Meditation and the color violet stimulate this chakra.

Affirmation: I release all my fears and doubts to the universe so that I can focus on the blessings in my life.

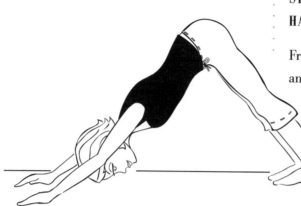

DOWN DOG

Start from your hands and knees, arms shoulder-width apart and extended in front of you, palms pressed into the floor.

Inhale: Standing on the balls of your feet, lift your hips toward the ceiling and straighten your arms and legs, rising up on your toes. Tuck your chin to your chest. Pause and take a few breaths here.

Exhale: Lower to the balls of your feet. Take a few breaths and work toward pressing both heels to the floor.

STANDING FORWARD FOLD, HANDS ON FLOOR

From Down Dog, walk your feet to your hands and stand up.

Inhale: Raise your arms out to the side, palms facing up, and reach up until your fingertips touch.

Exhale: Float your arms out to the side, palms facing down, bending forward from the waist, knees slightly bent. Touch the floor with your fingertips or, if you are flexible enough, the entire palm of your hand. Straighten your legs slowly.

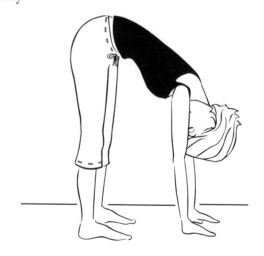

STANDING ARM RAISE

Inhale: Roll up slowly, raising your arms up overhead.

MOUNTAIN POSE

Exhale: Lower your arms to your sides. Roll your shoulders back to lift your chest, arms at your sides with the palms facing your body. Stand tall with your feet hip-width apart. Distribute your weight evenly over both feet, tuck your tailbone, and contract your abdomen. Visualize yourself as a strong, stable mountain.

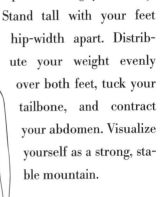

EXPRESS YOURSELF:
JOURNALING

Seeing life from a different perspective and thinking about yourself in new ways is an exciting part of yoga practice. Writing down your thoughts and feelings before and after yoga practice is a great way to search your soul, express your creativity, and generally ponder life's mysteries. Sometimes her journal is a girl's best friend.

Yoga Chick Tips

Establish a journaling style. Do you enjoy the weight of a pen in your hand and inky words unfolding on pristine paper? If so, invest in a nice, fat journal with widely spaced lined paper and a pen that fits comfortably in your hand. Or do your thoughts come faster than your hand can write? In that case, perhaps you need to write on your computer.

Write a few words after every yoga practice. Keep your journal handy so that you can make notes immediately following your session. Observe how your body felt before and after practice. Jotting down even a few sentence fragments after each practice will give your journal continuity over several months.

Make journaling a ritual. You may think it's indulgent to spend time on your journal, but consider it necessary to your mental health and personal growth. Make an agreement with yourself to set aside a specific time each week to write in your journal. Find a quiet place where you can curl up comfortably and be alone with your thoughts.

Warm-up Exercises to Break Through the Toughest Writer's Block

Breathe your way to inspiration. Our minds work best when they are calm and our bodies are relaxed. Close your eyes and concentrate on your breathing for one minute. Breathe normally and focus all your attention on the sound of every inhale and exhale. Imagine that you are inhaling inspiration and it is igniting your creativity like a spark to kindling.

Get in touch with your body. Getting in touch with how your body feels will help you understand its influence over other areas of your life. This insight can help you adjust your habits so that you feel in top physical condition more often. Close your eyes and conduct a body survey. Starting at the top, note how your head feels. Is it achy or light? How does your neck feel? Is it sore and tight? Can you feel stress lodged between your shoulder blades? Is that a cold virus tickling your throat or are you thirsty? Continue with your body survey until you have a good sense of how your body feels. Turning to your journal, draw a picture of yourself that reflects how your body feels. If your body feels light and energetic, you might draw a body with outstretched arms and feet that do not touch the ground. Write a few words that describe how your body feels today.

Get in touch with your emotions. Emotions can be powerful, but we grant some of them more power than others. Examining your emotions unravels their mystery and defuses their power. Pick one word that best describes how you feel emotionally: happy, joyful, excited, energetic, sad, depressed, cranky, neutral, etc. Is your emotion animal, vegetable, or mineral? How old is it? What color is it? What does it eat and drink to sustain itself? Will it live a long life or will it survive only a few minutes? Who are its allies and enemies? Is this emotion strong or weak? Powerful or a wimp? Do you like this emotion? Where does this emotion get its power? What tools do you have in your arsenal to tame this emotion?

Be present. We think of change as a dramatic event, but most of the change in our lives goes undetected because it is subtle and slow moving. This exercise uses an apple to help us cultivate a sharp eye and awareness of the present. Place a bright and shiny apple where you can easily see it. Study the apple and begin to write about what you see. What color is the apple? How big is it? Does it reflect light? Can you smell the apple? When you have exhausted every possible description of the apple, take a big bite. Take two big bites if you are hungry. What colors do you see now? Continue to study the apple and write about how it has changed. What do you see now? How does the apple taste and smell? How has its shape changed? Continue to study and write until you have finished eating the apple.

OM TO GO

Make each day count by living fully in the moment. Stay present to all the wonders that surround you.

CHAPTER FIVE

Take a Yoga Break

Renew your energy and get the kinks out after a hectic day.

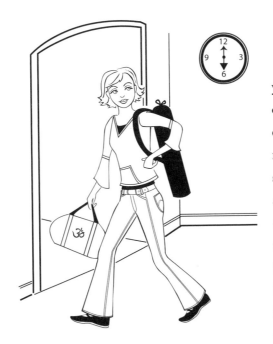

If a midafternoon energy dip makes you feel like a deflated balloon, you are not alone. Throughout the day, your energy ebbs and flows in a natural cycle. The afternoon doldrums leave many people feeling mentally flat and tired. Our bodies can work only so hard and our minds can process only so much information before they are overwhelmed. Curling up for a nap is tempting, but learning how to renew your energy will see you through a long night filled with activities, family, and friends.

This yoga practice gives you the chance to take a complete break from the day. Quieting your mind relieves your brain with some downtime, and doing a vigorous breathing exercise like Breath of Fire revs up your energy by pumping oxygen through the bloodstream and increasing your heart rate. Energy produces heat, and the effort required for Breath of Fire will warm you up in preparation for yoga practice. It is also a demanding ab workout!

Hunching over a desk all day and hauling an

overflowing bag has probably left you stiff, too. If losing the load is not an option, do this yoga practice to strengthen and stretch your spine. Your back will love you!

Your brain is a high-performance machine, and eating several small meals a day will keep its operating system humming. With a little planning, these energy-boosting practices will satisfy your brain and your appetite until it's time for dinner.

This practice generates energy by progressing through increasingly demanding poses. Stay with your breath and pay close attention to how your body responds to each pose.

BREATHE DEEPLY: BREATH OF FIRE

Whenever you need a quick pick-me-up, breathe fire. This breathing exercise powers up your energy by forcefully circulating oxygen through your system. Your body consumes oxygen, just as a car consumes fuel, to generate energy. Heat is a by-product of energy production, so expect to get nice and warm breathing fire!

1. Sit comfortably and inhale.
2. Contract your abdomen hard and fast to force air from your lungs.
3. Release your abdomen and you will inhale automatically.

The key to sustaining Breath of Fire is to focus on a loud exhalation. Like fire that makes a whooshing sound when it roars, your exhalation should make noise. Your lungs will naturally inhale, leaving you to concentrate on forcefully contracting your abdomen to exhale.

Practice 10 breaths at a time. You may get a little dizzy or light-headed, but this will pass as your brain becomes accustomed to the flood of oxygen. Work your way up to three sets of 10 or 20 breaths.

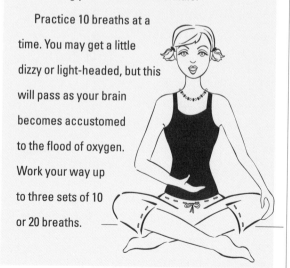

MOUNTAIN POSE

Stand tall with your feet hip-width apart. Roll your shoulders back, arms at your sides with the palms facing your body and fingers pointed to the floor. To get grounded, distribute your weight evenly over both feet. Feel all four corners of your feet on the ground. Raise and lower your toes a few times to check your stability. Tuck your tailbone, contract your abdomen, and extend your head from your neck for a nice, long spine. Look straight ahead or gaze down your nose. Visualize yourself as a strong and stable mountain and begin to focus on your breathing.

STANDING ARM RAISE WITH BACK BEND

Inhale: Raise your arms out to the sides of your body and reach up over your head, fingertips touching. Raise your chin to look up at your hands and continue to reach toward the ceiling, feeling your spine lengthen. When you feel stable and comfortable, bend back from the waist.

Exhale: Lower your arms to your sides and straighten your head and back.

As you become more flexible, work toward deepening your back bend. Visualize the crown of your head leading your back farther.

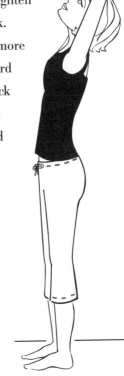

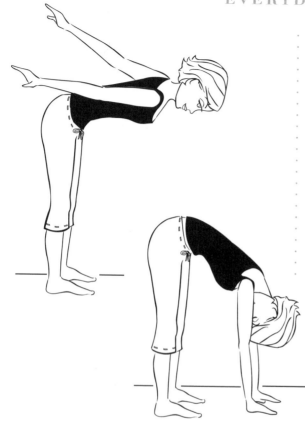

from the waist. Touch the floor with the palms of your hands, bending your knees if necessary.

Stay in this position for a few breaths. With each exhalation, shift your weight forward to the balls of your feet and bend a little deeper.

DOG AND CAT POSE

Starting from all fours, place your hands firmly on the floor directly below your shoulders, arms straight.

Inhale: Lift your chin and chest, bend your head back, lift your tailbone, and lower your back as deeply as you can.

STANDING FORWARD FOLD, HANDS ON FLOOR, WITH A SWAN DIVE

Inhale: Raise your arms out to the sides of your body and reach up over your head. Reach toward the ceiling, feeling your spine lengthen.

Exhale: Like a swan, gracefully float your arms out to the side, palms facing down, bending forward

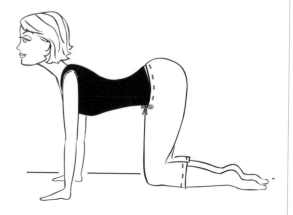

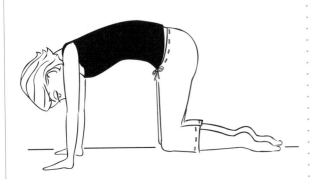

Exhale: Carefully tuck your chin to your chest, contract your abdominal muscles, and round your back.

Repeat this sequence several times, using your breath to create a comfortable rhythm.

SWEET DREAMS

Can't get to sleep? Do you crawl into bed, only to toss and turn? Everyone experiences insomnia once in a while, but if you have a hard time getting to sleep frequently, it's time to take action. Your body needs enough sleep to recover from its labors and renew its energy to start all over again the next day. Programmed to cycle with nature's rhythms of sunrise and sunset, your body gets confused when this cycle is interrupted. Continued sleep deprivation compromises your immune system, which means you will catch colds and flu more often, and it inhibits your physical performance in dance, sports, or yoga. Too little sleep affects your brain, too. Fatigue increases the production of the stress hormones that cause you to gain weight and become depressed. A few nights of tossing and turning can make a grouch out of anyone, even putting a strain on your relationships with friends and family.

But the good news is, you can develop better sleep habits if you know what's keeping you awake.

1. Examine your state of mind. Anxiety, worry, anticipation, excitement, frustration, self-doubt, and fear are just the beginning of a long list of emotions that stimulate the production of adrenaline, preventing you from falling asleep.

2. Examine what you eat and drink. Caffeine, sugar, and what you eat for dinner can create chemical havoc that affects your sleep patterns.

3. Examine your sleeping environment. An uncomfortable bed or a room that is too hot or too cold can distract you from falling asleep.

4. Examine your bedtime ritual. Do you do your homework, read for hours, or talk on the phone from bed?

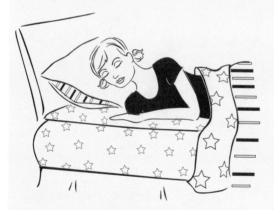

Try these proven techniques to take back your sweet dreams!

Eliminate caffeine from your life. Your body may be exhausted, but your mind is racing, fueled by a caf-

feine buzz. Cola, coffee, chocolate, some nutrition bars, and some sports drinks and vitamin-enhanced drinks are caffeinated, so read the labels. If you must have caffeine, drink it before 2 p.m.

Turn your mind toward sleep. It's hard to turn off those uncontrollable racing thoughts that keep us up at night. (For more information about how to quiet your mind, see "The Power of Sitting Still: Meditation" on page 74.) The following visualization exercise focuses your thoughts on sleep: Lie comfortably on your back and breathe normally. Imagine yourself on a beach, sitting near the water's edge, looking out to the horizon. Sleep is on the horizon and you want to get there. In your imagination, listen to the waves lapping against the shoreline. Tune in to the rhythm of the waves coming in and then receding from the beach. Coordinate your breath with the waves. Exhale as the waves recede from the beach. With each exhalation, let go of your body and think of sleep.

Create a bedtime ritual. A good bedtime routine includes things like a little downtime to unwind before you climb into bed. A good routine supports healthy sleeping habits. The first step is getting yourself in the mood to sleep. Make it a habit to go to bed and wake up at the same times each day. Over time, your body will adjust to this pattern and automatically begin to shut down right around bedtime.

Create a transition between your evening activities and your bedtime ritual by taking a warm bath or shower. A small cup of warm milk contains tryptophan, a chemical that will make you sleepy. (Avoid chocolate milk; it contains caffeine.) You also could try a cup of chamomile tea.

The second step in your bedtime ritual relaxes your body and your mind. Practice one or two restful yoga poses in your room. A seated twist and Child's Pose are good starters, but you may prefer other poses.

After yoga, climb into bed and turn off the light. Lie on your back and breathe naturally. Focus on your body. Visualize your body full of sand. Starting at your feet, imagine the sand is slowly leaking from your toes. Let go of your feet as you feel them sink into the bed. As the sand leaks from your legs,

let go. Let your legs sink into the bed. Continue up your body, visualizing the sand leaking from your torso, your arms, your neck, and finally your head.

Don't fight sleep. Sink into it and enjoy sweet dreams.

STANDING, HANDS CLASPED BEHIND BACK

Stand with feet slightly apart and clasp your hands behind your back, arms straight and pointing down.

Inhale: Roll your shoulders up and back. Hold this pose for three to five breaths.

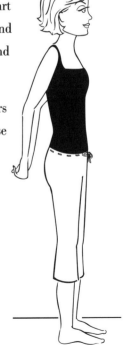

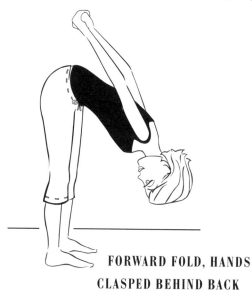

**FORWARD FOLD, HANDS
CLASPED BEHIND BACK**

Exhale: Lift your arms a few inches away from your body and bend forward from the waist into a forward fold. To increase the stretch, raise your arms a little higher. Hold this pose for three to five breaths.

WARRIOR II

Start from a standing pose and jump your legs about three or four feet apart. Point your right foot out 90 degrees and pivot your left foot in about 45 degrees. Raise your arms to shoulder height and stretch out to the sides, palms facing the floor.

Inhale: Turn your head to the left and slowly bend your left knee until your thigh is parallel to the ground. Keep your knee right over the ankle. Focus your gaze on the middle finger of your left hand. Hold this pose for three to five breaths.

Pivot your feet to turn to the opposite side and repeat.

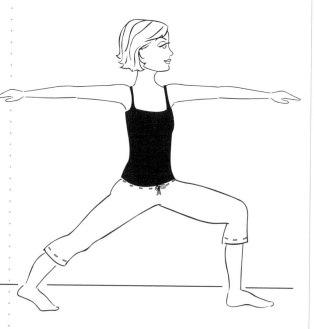

TRIANGLE

Start from Warrior II stance with legs wide, left foot turned out 90 degrees and right foot turned in 45 degrees, arms stretched out to your sides.

Inhale: Turn your head to the left and reach out with your left arm.

Exhale: Bend to the left from your waist to touch your left ankle with your left hand. Raise your right arm straight up and look up at your right hand. If this position hurts your neck, look at the floor. Stay in this position for three to five breaths.

Pivot on your feet to repeat on the opposite side.

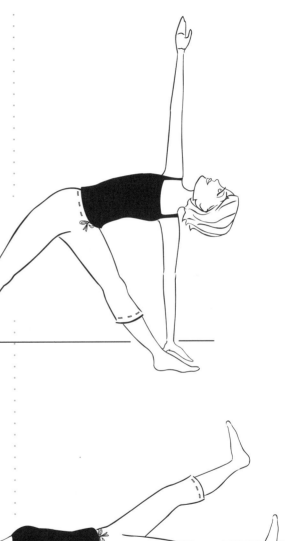

LEG LIFT

Lie on your back, legs together and arms at your sides, palms facing down. Take a deep breath.

Exhale: Contract your lower abdomen and raise one leg a few inches from the floor. Hold this pose for three to five slow, even breaths.

Repeat on the opposite side.

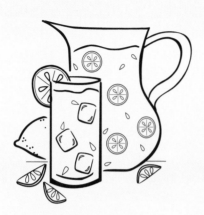

- A half bagel topped with one slice of cheddar or Swiss cheese.
- A piece of whole wheat bread topped with a sliced hard-boiled egg.
- One cup of cottage cheese with fruit.
- Celery sticks spread with cream cheese.

SNACK ATTACK

Before reaching for a sugary, caffeinated beverage—and the energy spike and crash that come with it—try a snack with staying power. The citrus in this spritzer will give you a mental boost, and a protein-and-carbohydrate snack provides enough slow-burning fuel to keep you up and running through dinner.

Smart Snacks

- A sliced apple spread with one or two tablespoons of peanut butter.

CITRUS SPRITZER

1-inch piece fresh gingerroot, peeled and
coarsely chopped
1 cup boiling water
2 tablespoons lemon juice
2 tablespoons lime juice
2 tablespoons honey, stevia, or Splenda
pinch of salt
1 cup sparkling water

Steep the ginger in the boiling water for five minutes. Strain out the ginger and add the lemon and lime juices, honey, and salt. Cool.

Add sparkling water and serve on ice.

Makes 2 servings.

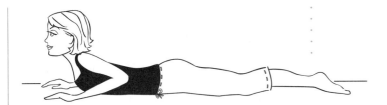

HALF COBRA

Lie on your stomach with your legs about one foot apart and the tops of your feet flat on the floor. Place your forearms on the floor with your hands just below your shoulders.

Inhale: Resting on your forearms, use your shoulders and upper back muscles to lift your head, neck, and shoulders from the floor. Look straight ahead. Hold this pose for three to five breaths.

FULL COBRA

Inhale: Straighten your arms as you lift your head and chest from the floor. Look straight ahead. Hold this pose for three to five breaths.

PRONE SPIRAL TWIST

Lie on your back, knees pulled into your chest. Use your hand to roll your knees

to the left until they touch the floor. Spread your arms out to the sides and look to the right. Hold this pose for a few breaths.

Pivot your knees to repeat on the opposite side.

WHAT'S YOUR DOSHA?

If milk makes you gag and you crave salad greens, your Kapha could be out of balance. It's hard to feel healthy and grounded when your doshas are doing somersaults.

In Ayurveda, the Indian practice of medicine, every person is born with a specific physical and mental constitution made up of a unique combination of doshas—Pitta, Vata, and Kapha. Each dosha is associated with an element—Vata with air, Pitta with fire, and Kapha with the earth. One dosha usually dominates your health and your personality, shaping your strengths and your quirks.

Health is a balanced dosha system and things such as stress, fatigue, and a poor diet can throw your doshas out of balance, leaving you vulnerable to aches and pains, roller-coaster moods, or worse.

The first step toward keeping yourself in balance is understanding your dosha. Certain foods and exercises are compatible with each dosha, and the wrong food can aggravate it. For example, Pitta-dominated people are nervous and high-strung, and yoga practice and comfort foods like oatmeal and mangoes can help keep them calm.

Answer the following questions and add up your score to determine your dosha.

First, determine your physical build.

❏ I am light and delicate. My wrists and ankles are small in proportion to my size, and my legs and arms are long. I may be very short or very tall. I look slender and willowy, perhaps like a dancer. (1 point)

❏ I am medium. My wrists and ankles are in proportion to my size. My body is nicely toned, my height is average, and my weight is right for my size. (2 points)

❏ I am solid. My wrists and ankles are thick. I am tall and large. My body appears strong and powerful, though I do not have much muscle tone. I am not very active. Sometimes I feel a little clumsy. (3 points)

What is your skin like?

❏ My skin tone is olive or darker. I get a nice tan. My skin does tend to be dry. Sometimes I get flaky stuff on my face. (1 point)

❏ My skin tone is fair, and my skin is soft. I break out once in a while. I have freckles, too. (2 points)

❏ My skin tone is pale, but my cheeks are really rosy sometimes. My skin is oily, and I break out fairly often. (3 points)

And your teeth?

❏ My teeth are small, sharp, and white. (1 point)

❏ My teeth are medium and white. (2 points)

❏ My teeth are large and yellowish. (3 points)

What are your lips like?

❏ My lips are thin and get dry sometimes. I use a lot of lip conditioner. (1 point)

❏ My lips are soft and pink. Usually I use gloss to make them bright. (2 points)

❏ My lips are full and dark pink. I don't wear anything on my lips. (3 points)

How are your fingernails?

❏ Yuck, short and brittle. My fingernail polish is always chipped. (1 point)

❏ They are soft and don't break easily. I don't wear fingernail polish. (2 points)

❏ My nails grow fast and are hard. (3 points)

What is your hair like?

❏ Taming my hair is a battle. It is fine and curly—or it is coarse and kinky. Either way, it's unmanageable. (1 point)

❏ Don't hate me—I am blessed with great, medium-bodied, manageable hair. (2 points)

❏ My hair is like a horse's mane—full, thick, and wavy. (3 points)

How is your face shaped?

❏ My face is long and has sharp angles. My nose is small, though. (1 point)

❏ My face is round and my cheeks are full and rosy. I have strong features. (2 points)

❏ My face is shaped like a heart, my chin is pointy, and my nose is pert. (3 points)

How well do you sleep?

❏ I have a hard time getting to sleep and am restless and wake up often during the night. I often wake up feeling tired and cranky. (1 point)

❏ I fall asleep easily and sleep through the night. I wake up and often remember my dreams. I usually feel refreshed after a good night's sleep. (2 points)

❏ I sleep like a rock. I don't think I dream. At least I don't remember my dreams. (3 points)

How do you behave in conversations with your friends?

❏ Forget about trying to get a word in edgewise if you're talking to me. I'm a fast talker. And I just keep right on talking. (1 point)

❏ I'm in training to be a broadcast personality. I am very confident and am well spoken. (2 points)

❏ Sometimes I have a hard time getting right to the point. It takes me some time to express my thoughts in conversation. (3 points)

How would you describe your biggest emotional flaw?

❏ I'm a meltdown waiting to happen. (1 point)

❏ I can barely keep a lid on my temper. (2 points)

❏ I cling possessively to people I like. (3 points)

Add up your score. If your score is 10–16, your dominant dosha is Vata. If your score is 17–23, your dominant dosha is Pitta. If your score is 24–30, your dominant dosha is Kapha.

About Vata Dosha

If you are the first one to raise your hand to volunteer for a school project and later attend only half the meetings, you could be a Vata. Active, restless, enthusiastic, creative, and a little flaky sometimes, Vatas are very tall or very short, with long face and small, narrow noses that reflect their thin build. Vatas enjoy a wide circle of acquaintances, but few deep friendships. Vatas love to shop, so watch your budget.

About Pitta Dosha

Do people call you a natural leader? Then you must be a Pitta. Ambitious Pitta is quick and alert, an articulate speaker and confident in the spotlight. Pittas are moderately built with naturally toned muscles. They usually have soft, fair skin and a heart-shaped face with soft features. Pittas often are on best-dressed lists because they save their spending money for little luxuries like clothes.

About Kapha Dosha

If you are an earth mother type, you could very well be a Kapha. Caring and compassionate, grounded and patient, Kaphas are rocks of stability. Kaphas are a little too content sometimes and become lethargic and need a lot of sleep. Kaphas often are large people, with thick and wavy hair and a full face.

To keep your doshas balanced, eat and exercise as follows:

COMPATIBLE FOODS

VATA — Sweet, sour, and salty. You can start your day with oatmeal or smoothies made with whole milk and rich fruits like bananas, mangoes, or figs. Stick to simple yet filling meals, such as grilled chicken breast with a side of roasted root vegetables like beets or carrots, along with whole grain rice seasoned with cumin or coriander.

PITTA — Sweet, bitter, and astringent. Enjoy a breakfast of whole grain cereal with sliced sweet apples or berries, and milk. Stick to low-fat meals, such as firm whitefish with potatoes or squash, and steamed asparagus or broccoli drizzled with a little ghee (clarified butter). Snack on sunflower seeds.

KAPHA — Pungent, bitter, and astringent. Indulge in a wide range of grains, like oats, muesli, and couscous, topped with cranberries, pomegranates, or dried fruits. Limit your dairy to one glass of milk a day. Top a colorful salad composed of leafy greens with shrimp. Snack on almonds and walnuts in moderation.

COMPATIBLE EXERCISE

VATA

Maintain your flexibility, strength, and balance by practicing Flow yoga. Vigorous walking can provide a good aerobic workout and will help you burn off excess energy.

PITTA

Maintain your strength, flexibility, and balance by practicing Ashtanga yoga. Engage in a variety of activities that you can do with other people, such as group jogging, cycling, and team sports like volleyball.

KAPHA

Maintain your strength, flexibility and balance by practicing Bikram yoga. Kapha benefits from vigorous exercise, like running and weight lifting.

RABBIT

Kneel on the floor with your feet together and your knees wide apart. Sit back on your heels. Bend forward from your waist and place your forehead on the floor. Round your back and reach back to clasp the heels of your feet.

Inhale: Pull on your heels until you feel a gentle stretch in your back.

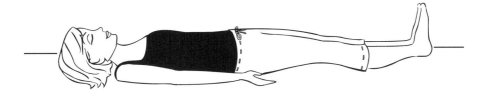

PEACEFUL POSE

Lie flat on your back on the floor with your arms and legs open a comfortable distance apart. Breathe naturally.

OM TO GO

Use the power of your imagination every day to visualize your dreams, setting daily goals that will help you reach them.

CHAPTER SIX

Welcome the Weekend

Let the practice inspire you!

Ah, the weekend! Finally you've got the time for a full yoga practice that works your body and your mind. Power up your Victory Breathing technique for this demanding sequence of yoga poses. The Warrior sequence will challenge you out of your physical and mental comfort zone. Channeling the energy and light of the sun in Sun Salutations will give you inspiration for the rest of the weekend. Strong abdominal muscles support strength and bal-ance, and these poses draw their energy from a strong core body. This practice will challenge you, for sure, but it will reward you with well-toned thighs, arms, and abs, as well as a newfound sense of courage and determination.

Challenge and stress build physical muscles and mental resilience. The Warrior poses tone thighs and hips by creating isometric tension in your leg muscles. Warrior also represents the balance between effort, concentration, and surrender that you need to achieve results, both on the mat and in life. When you stay in familiar territory and your body and mind can cruise on autopilot, your attention can wander and your yoga practice stays the same. A lot like life. The way you grow, change, and move forward to the next level in any situation is by setting goals and pushing toward them. It takes a lot of concentration and self-discipline to manage tough projects and extra activities.

The way you react to challenging situations determines what you get from life. Practice self-observation as you hold Warrior for several breaths: Do you give up easily, pulling out of the pose at the first sign of discomfort in your legs? Is your mind focused on your breathing or is it listening to your critical internal voice?

If you find the pose challenging, try something different. Use your breath to relax into the pose and see what happens. Let your leg muscles soften. Visualize your breath massaging your thighs. A small shift in how you respond to a challenge sometimes can create a big change in the outcome. The next time you are in a tough spot, summon your inner Warrior for strength, persistence, and flexibility!

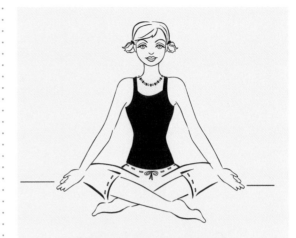

BREATHE DEEPLY: VICTORY BREATH

This is an advanced breathing technique that gives you more control over your breath. The noise you make should sound like what you hear when you put a seashell to your ear—the soft echo of the rush and roar of the ocean. Use your Victory Breath to channel energy where you need it during challenging yoga poses.

1. Begin by breathing slowly and deeply through your nose.

2. Constrict the back of your throat just a little.

3. Contract your abdomen and exhale.

Sun Salutations are a classic series of flow poses that link body, mind, spirit, and breath, and are one of the oldest series of yoga poses, dating back to a time when the sun was the primary source of light. The series is the warm-up for this practice, and you can honor an ancient tradition and channel the sun's energy by practicing your Sun Salutations early in the morning, facing east as the sun rises on the horizon.

After all this work, your body is going to need some TLC. Slip into a steaming bathtub filled with soothing natural mineral salts, lean back, and consider how this yoga practice has inspired you! Relax.

This demanding practice channels your energy and focus. If you begin to lose control of a pose, detach from the discomfort and focus on your Victory Breathing. Avoid the instinct to use your brute strength and tighten up. When we try to control things, we get rigid, and change can happen only if you are open to it. So soften up your legs a little, and focus on five full breaths.

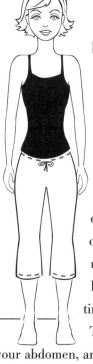

MOUNTAIN POSE

Stand tall with your feet hip-width apart. Roll your shoulders back, arms at your sides with the palms facing your body and fingers pointed to the floor. To get grounded, distribute your weight evenly over both feet. Feel all four corners of your feet on the ground. Raise and lower your toes a few times to check your stability. Tuck your tailbone, contract your abdomen, and extend your head from your neck for a nice long spine. Look straight ahead or gaze down your nose.

Inhale: Start Victory Breathing. Once you feel centered and connected to your breath, begin your yoga practice.

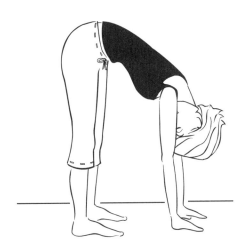

STANDING ARM RAISE WITH A BACK BEND

Inhale: Raise your arms out to the sides of your body and reach up over your head, fingertips touching. Raise your chin to look up at your hands and continue to reach toward the ceiling, feeling your spine lengthen. When you feel stable and comfortable, bend back from the waist.

Exhale: Lower your arms and straighten your head and back.

STANDING FORWARD FOLD, HANDS ON FLOOR

Inhale: Raise your arms out to the sides of your body and reach up over your head. Continue to reach toward the ceiling, feeling your spine lengthen.

Exhale: Tuck your chin to your chest, bend forward from your waist, arms out to the side, palms facing down. Gracefully bend forward and touch the floor with the palms of your hands. Bend your knees if you need to.

Stay in this position for a few breaths. With each exhalation, shift your weight forward to the balls of your feet and bend a little deeper.

RIGHT LEG LUNGE

Inhale: From a standing position, step your right foot forward and bend your right leg at the knee making sure that your knee does not extend farther forward than your right ankle. Place your hands on the floor on either side of your right foot for support and step your left leg back.

Exhale: Rise, raising your arms above your head if you can. You should feel a gentle stretch in the front of your left hip.

Variation: You may leave your hands on your knee for support.

Return your hands to the floor, hands on either side of your foot. Step your left leg forward to meet your right leg and move to your hands and knees.

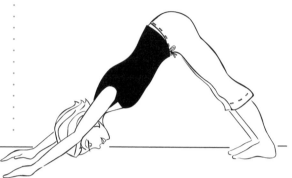

DOWN DOG

Inhale: Straighten your arms, press your palms into the floor, tuck your chin to your chest, and push your hips high up in the air. Straighten your knees and push your heels toward the floor.

Stay in this pose for a few breaths.

Bend your knees to the floor, then lower the rest of your body to the floor.

COBRA

Rise up on your forearms, hands just below your shoulders.

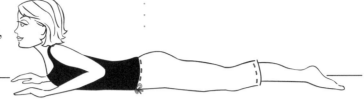

Inhale: Resting on your forearms, use your shoulders and upper back muscles to lift your head, neck, and shoulders from the floor. Look straight ahead. Hold this pose for three to five breaths.

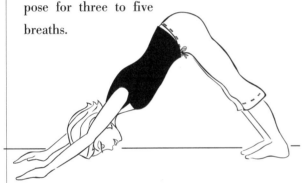

DOWN DOG

Start from your hands and knees.

Inhale: Straighten your arms, press your palms into the floor, tuck your chin to your chest, and push your hips high up in the air. Straighten your knees and push your heels toward the floor. Stay in this pose for a few breaths.

LEFT LEG LUNGE

Inhale: Move your left leg forward, bent at the knee, and place your hands on the floor on either side of your left foot. Make sure your left knee does not extend farther forward than your left ankle. Step your right leg back.

Exhale: Rise, raising your arms above your head if you can. Feel a gentle stretch in the front of your right hip.

Inhale: Return your hands to the floor, hands on either side of your left foot, and bring yourself to a standing position.

STANDING FORWARD FOLD, HANDS ON FLOOR

Inhale: Raise your arms out to the sides of your body and reach up over your head. Continue to reach toward the ceiling, feeling your spine lengthen.

Exhale: Tuck your chin to your chest, bend forward from your waist, arms out to the side, palms facing down, hands to the floor. Stay in this position for a few breaths.

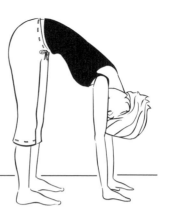

STANDING ARM RAISE WITH BACK BEND

Inhale: Raise your arms out to the sides of your body and reach up over your head, fingertips touching. Continue to reach toward the ceiling, feeling your spine lengthen. When you feel stable and comfortable, bend back from the waist.

Exhale: Lower your arms and straighten your head and back.

MOUNTAIN POSE

Pause here to reconnect with your breath in Mountain Pose. Focus on your Victory Breath. Once you feel centered and connected to your breath, move on to the next pose.

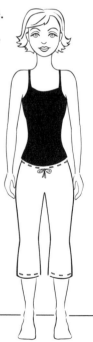

WARRIOR II

Jump your feet three to four feet apart. Point your right foot out 90 degrees and pivot your left foot in about 45 degrees. Raise your arms to shoulder height and stretch them out to the sides, palms facing the floor.

Inhale: Turn your head to the left and slowly bend your left knee until your thigh is parallel to the ground. Keep your knee right over the ankle. Focus your gaze on the middle finger of your left hand for three to five breaths.

Pivot your feet and repeat on the opposite side.

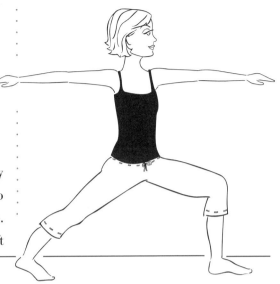

EXTENDED SIDE ANGLE

Start from Warrior II pose, left knee bent.

Exhale: With your left arm reaching out, bend from your waist to the left, placing your fingertips or entire hand on or next to your left foot.

Inhale: Raise your right arm straight up over your head. Look up.

Exhale: Rise to standing. Repeat Warrior II and Extended Side Angle on the right side.

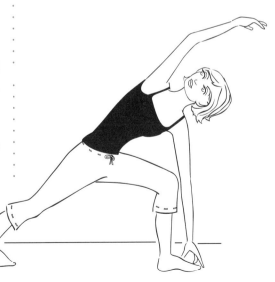

CORE FUSION: STRENGTH, COURAGE AND WISDOM

Strong abdominal muscles—or a strong core—nourish the third chakra, the source of your strength, courage, and wisdom. The third chakra begins to project its strongest energetic influence during adolescence, a time in life when girls start to think for themselves and make decisions independent of their family and friends. With life experience comes an increase in self-confidence that gives voice to your gut instincts. With your ears tuned in to your inner voice, you begin to trust yourself and your abilities. As you develop your individuality, you learn your strengths and weaknesses. If you trust your abilities, you will take risks. If you have self-confidence, you will have the courage to do the right thing, even when you must act alone and apart from your friends. Sticking to your truest beliefs develops integrity, but only after you examine those beliefs. Our beliefs sometimes change as we gain more life experience. Wisdom develops when you accept who you are and can move forward in life with self-respect.

Yoga Chicks work those abdominal muscles for strength, courage, and wisdom!

TREE

Stand tall and steady and gaze at a fixed object.

Inhale: Use your right hand to guide your right foot to the inside of your left leg, either above or below the knee—but not directly on the knee. Steady yourself and raise your hands above your head. Stay in this pose for a few breaths.

Release your foot and repeat on opposite side.

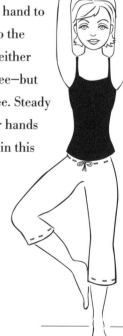

WARRIOR III

Inhale: Raise your arms out to your sides at shoulder height and maintain your gaze on the floor a few feet in front of you.

Exhale: Step forward onto your right leg, get your balance, and then bend forward from your waist, lifting your left leg up and straight out behind you.

Inhale: If you can, bring your arms together in front of you.

Release and repeat on the opposite side.

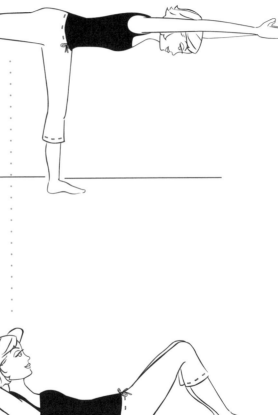

CRUNCH

Lie on your back with your knees bent, feet planted firmly on the floor, arms behind your head, gently supporting your neck. Take a deep breath.

Exhale: Contract your abdomen and lift your shoulders from the floor a few inches.

Repeat this sequence twelve times.

BIKE WITH LEG EXTENSION

Take a deep breath.

Exhale: Contract your abdomen and lift your shoulders from the floor a few inches while reaching your left leg out as if you were riding a bicycle.

Inhale: Let your knees meet in the middle and extend your right leg, continuing to contract your abdomen.

Repeat this sequence twelve times.

BIKE WITH A TWIST FROM THE WAIST

Take a deep breath.

Exhale: Lift your right shoulder from the floor and twist it across your body to your left knee. At the same time, reach your right leg out as if you were riding a bicycle.

Inhale: Let your knees meet in the middle and extend your left leg, continuing to contract your abdomen while you twist your left shoulder to your right knee.

Repeat this sequence twelve times.

BOW

Turn over to lie on your stomach, knees bent, feet flexed. Reach around and clasp your ankles.

Inhale: Raise your head, shoulders, and chest from the ground.

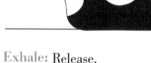

Exhale: Release.

Repeat three times.

SEATED TWIST

Sit on the floor with your legs extended. Raise your left leg with knee bent and place your left foot on the outside of your right knee. Anchor your left hand on the floor behind you for stability and place your right elbow on the outside of your left knee. Twist gently to your left as you exhale. Hold this pose for a few breaths.

   Repeat on the opposite side.

PEACEFUL POSE

Lie flat on your back on the floor with your arms and legs open a comfortable distance apart, but no more than a few inches. Breathe naturally.

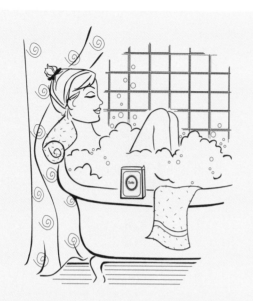

SPA TREATMENT

It's time to rejuvenate! The earliest spas were remote oases located near natural mineral springs and thermal waters. People traveled long distances to sweat out toxins in the roiling, steamy waters. Contemporary spas offer a wide range of treatments to restore inner and outer radiance. With the right ingredients, you can transform your own bathroom into an oasis and replenish your healthy glow.

Mineral Salts Bath

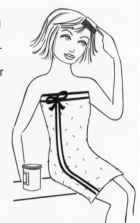

Head off post-yoga practice aches in a bath. Pour two cups of Epsom salts into a hot steamy bath, dip below the water, and soak. Use the remaining salts by the handful to exfoliate your feet.

Super Smoothing Hair Conditioner

While you're soaking in the tub, condition the ends of your hair. Slather just the last few inches of your tresses with mayonnaise, wrap your hair in a towel, and relax. Wash your hair well. And be careful: The olive oil and egg yolks in real mayo will make your tub or shower slippery.

Treat Your Feet

In the East, the feet are the gateway to the body. The feet contain a delicate network of acupressure points that correspond to various organs, limbs, and other places on your body. Massage your feet using lots of lotion that contains tea tree

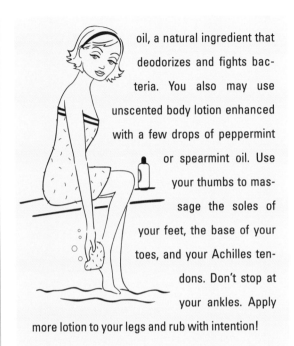

oil, a natural ingredient that deodorizes and fights bacteria. You also may use unscented body lotion enhanced with a few drops of peppermint or spearmint oil. Use your thumbs to massage the soles of your feet, the base of your toes, and your Achilles tendons. Don't stop at your ankles. Apply more lotion to your legs and rub with intention!

Eye Soothers

Homework, computers, air pollution, and allergies can make your eyes sore and puffy. Chill a fresh, fat cucumber in the freezer for ten minutes. Don't let it get frozen! Slice two thick rounds from the cuke, lie down in a comfortable position, and place the slices over your eyes. Breathe deeply and relax.

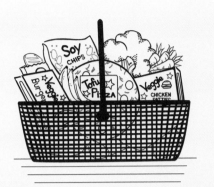

TO BE OR NOT TO BE
A VEGETARIAN

A long history links a vegetarian diet with yoga. Many yoginis believe a vegetarian diet is gentler on the body and the digestive system. Maintaining a plant-based diet allows them to eat in harmony with the cycles of nature. Some interpret the yoga concept of "do no harm" to mean it's morally wrong to kill animals.

Choosing to become a vegetarian is a personal choice, one that should not be made lightly. How you eat and what you eat today influences the future course of your health, appearance, energy level, athletic performance, intellectual ability, and mental outlook. Before changing your diet, get smart about your nutritional needs and how you will meet them through a vegetarian diet. Seek out a nutritionist who can help you with planning meals that include the right amount of protein, fat, iron, and calcium, the nutrients most often missing from vegetarian diets.

"Going Veggie": What Does This Mean?

"Vegetarian" means different things to different people. Vegetarian eating styles vary, too. Some people avoid only red meat and call themselves vegetarians. At the opposite end of the spectrum are people whose lifestyle is based on respect for all animal life. Does one of these labels fit your needs?

- "Everything but red meat" vegetarians avoid beef and other dark meat, but continue to consume chicken, fish, and shellfish.
- "Fish only" vegetarians avoid all red and white meats, but will eat fish and shellfish.
- "Lacto-ovo" vegetarians do not eat meat, poultry, or fish, but do eat all dairy products—milk, yogurt, cheese—and eggs and plant-based foods, like fruits, vegetables, beans, grains, and nuts.
- "Lacto" vegetarians eat milk, cheese, and yogurt, but refuse eggs or any foods that contain eggs.
- A "fruitarian" eats only fresh fruit and some vegetables such as cucumbers, tomatoes, squashes, and avocados.
- "Raw food" vegetarians believe cooking food destroys important enzymes that our bodies need for peak health. They eat raw whole fruits, vegetables, nuts, seeds, beans, and grains. A variation on the raw food diet is the raw living-foods diet. To preserve nutritious enzymes contained in raw foods, they can be warmed to only 115 degrees.
- Vegans (pronounced *vee-guns*) eat only plant-based foods. What separates vegans from pure vegetarians is their commitment to animals and the natural ecology of the Earth. They do not use leather, wool, or silk, or any other products that have been made from using animal parts.
- A "flexitarian" moves between eating styles,

usually without the guilt or remorse many vegetarians feel when they fall off the wagon to order a burger. Many flexitarians adopt an Ayurvedic-based approach to eating by varying their diet according to the season. A specific eating plan is determined by each individual's dosha, but it is not unusual for a flexitarian to go meatless in the spring as part of a cleansing ritual and reintroduce meat into their diet in the summer.

- "Vegetarian aware" eaters are more concerned about where and how animals are raised and how they are processed. These people look for organic, natural, and humanely raised products.

The Responsibilities of a Vegetarian Lifestyle

A well-planned vegetarian diet can be healthy and nutritionally sound, though it does take some planning. Protein and fat in meat fills you up and satisfies your appetite. You can reproduce the satisfied feeling you get from meat with bean- and grain-based products that are processed to look, feel, and taste like meat. Soy burgers and sausages are available in a variety of flavors and are substantial enough to satisfy a hungry appetite.

Pack in Protein

The risk of a protein shortfall in your diet is low if your vegetarian meal plan draws from a variety of foods, including protein-rich dairy products and eggs, dried beans, and whole grains. In Asian and Mediterranean cultures, meat is one of many ingredients used to season a dish based on a grain or vegetable, and it is easily eliminated with little impact on the finished dish. Look to these cultures for ideas to inspire your meal planning.

Eat Your Fruits and Veggies

It goes without saying; any meal plan must incorporate vegetables and fruits for fiber, vitamins, and minerals. Also, vegetables and fruit provide variety. Widen your horizons by sampling one new fruit or vegetable each week. Increasingly, specialty fruits and vegetables are available that will add new interest to everyday meals.

A Word about Organic and Natural Foods

Many people who are concerned about the quality of the food they eat are interested in organic. From the produce section to the frozen food case, almost every aisle in an average grocery store contains foods that are certified organic.

The goal of organic agriculture is to use materials and farming practices that preserve and protect a healthy, interdependent relationship between soil life, plants, animals, and humans. Organic food producers who comply with the standards set by the United States Department of Agriculture are entitled to use the "USDA Certified Organic" label.

Because organic foods are grown without pesticides and chemical fertilizers, they look different from conventionally grown produce. Organic fruits and vegetables may not be uniform in shape, size, and color. As with many things in life, though, don't judge organic produce by its cover. Most people find that organic fruits and vegetables taste more vibrant and unique than that of homogenous, conventionally grown products.

Many food producers label their products "all natural." Unlike the organic certification, there is no governing body that defines "natural." The natural label is a marketing creation that suggests a product has been minimally processed and is made of wholesome ingredients. The best way to know if a product meets this test is to read the ingredients label.

OM TO GO

It's not how many breaths you take, but how deeply each breath inspires you!

CHAPTER SEVEN

Striking a Balance

*When the pressure builds, turn to yoga for
that calm, peaceful feeling.*

Your day has left you feeling frazzled. You hardly made a dent in your to-do list, your best friend is acting funny, you still haven't picked up your mom's birthday present, and a stack of assignments is staring at you from your desk.

That tightness you feel in your chest is your body's stress-response system kicking in. Stress is a fact of life, but chronic stress stimulates your body to release a tidal wave of the stress hormone cortisol, which knocks your mind, body, and spirit out of balance. Headaches, stomachaches, and even asthma are common stress-related health problems. Muscles tighten up, creating back and neck pain, and it's hard to think straight.

A great way to recenter and release tension is to hit your yoga mat and focus on three proven stress management techniques: breathing, medi-

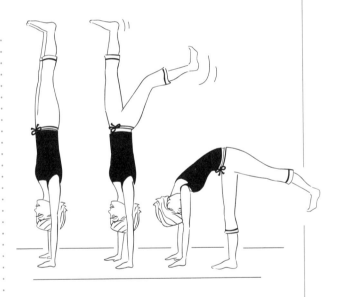

tation, and yoga poses that slow down your racing heart rate, soothe your mind, and release tension from your joints.

While stress gets a bad rap, it's not always a bad thing. Sometimes the stress of an approaching deadline can get the creative juices flowing. Stress is like a helium-filled balloon: too little gas and the balloon won't fly. Overfill it, and the balloon may burst. The challenge is in finding the right balance.

When stress overwhelms your ability to cope, you feel distressed. The difference between stress and distress is how much control you feel you have over the situation. People who feel as if they don't have control over their lives feel stressed out more often than those who feel in control. Sometimes the difference between feeling stressed and calm is letting go of the need to control a situation. Every person has a unique stress threshold, that place where they teeter between control and chaos. Stress management is recognizing that threshold and managing your response to a stressful situation.

Meditation takes practice, but it rewards you with better self-awareness about how you respond to stress. The smallest shift in your attitude toward a stressful situation can reduce its impact. If you view a challenging assignment as an opportunity to stretch yourself, the stress you feel will stimulate your creativity and energize your efforts.

This practice peaks in two dynamic balancing poses, Eagle and Dancer. These demanding poses teach us that balance is not a state of perfect stillness but a state of confident and graceful movement.

To maintain your balance, stare at a fixed object and press the foot of your standing leg firmly into the floor. It's okay to sway a little bit. Think of a graceful treetop swaying in the wind, held firmly in place by strong roots. The key to restoring your balance in yoga and life is getting right back up if you fall.

MOUNTAIN POSE

Stand tall with your feet hip-width apart. Roll your shoulders back, arms at your sides with the palms facing your body and fingers pointed to the floor. To get grounded, distribute your weight evenly over both feet. Feel all four corners of your feet on the ground. Raise and lower your toes a few times to check your stability. Tuck your tailbone, contract your abdomen, and extend your head from your neck for a nice, long spine. Look straight ahead or gaze down your nose.

Inhale: Start Victory Breathing (see page 55). When you feel centered and connected to your breath, begin your yoga practice.

STANDING ARM RAISE WITH A BACK BEND

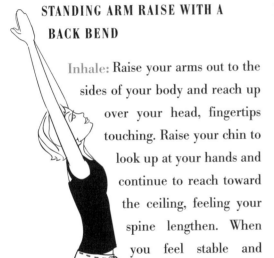

Inhale: Raise your arms out to the sides of your body and reach up over your head, fingertips touching. Raise your chin to look up at your hands and continue to reach toward the ceiling, feeling your spine lengthen. When you feel stable and comfortable, bend back from the waist.

Exhale: Lower your arms and straighten your head and back.

STANDING FORWARD FOLD, ARMS FOLDED

Stand tall and roll your shoulders back.

Inhale: Raise your arms out to the sides of your body and reach up over your head. Raise your chin to look up at your hands and continue to reach toward the ceiling, feeling your spine lengthen.

Exhale: Tuck your chin to your chest, bend forward from your waist, arms out to the side, palms facing down. Fold your arms one over the other, clasping your elbows. Bend your knees and point the crown of your head to the floor. Feel your lower back stretch. Stay in this position for a few breaths.

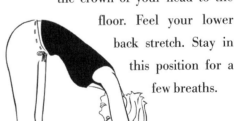

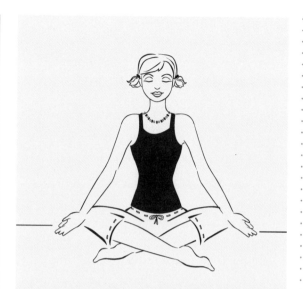

THE POWER OF SITTING STILL: MEDITATION

Meditation is a powerful mental process and central to the yoga lifestyle. Yoga Chicks meditate to develop concentration, patience, and insight—important tools on your yoga journey of self-discovery. Meditation requires little: all you have to do is clear your mind, sit quietly, and breathe. In return, it will leave you feeling clearheaded and calm. Simple, but not easy.

In yoga, the ongoing thoughts and chatter in your head are called monkey mind. Your mind automatically jumps from thought to thought like an impatient monkey moving from one tree branch to the next. Focusing on a single reference point, like the sound of your breath, a candle, or a chant, helps quiet the voices in your head and develops your powers of concentration.

Even when you successfully quiet your monkey mind, it is impossible to control the unexpected thoughts that pop up during meditation, like the long list of assignments sitting on your desk or the errand you promised to do for your friend. This is natural. It's easy to let these distracting thoughts frustrate you and interrupt your meditation practice. Sometimes, powerful thoughts will surface that upset you. Perhaps you have had an argument with your best friend and the thought of it makes you feel angry all over again. No matter how powerfully they tug at you, acknowledge your thoughts but let them continue to move through your mind without reacting or grabbing hold of them. Return to your breath. Wisdom comes from accepting that all your thoughts, pleasant and painful, are a natural part of being human. Be patient with yourself, and peace will come.

How to meditate:

1. Sit comfortably in a seated position in a quiet place. Use a blanket for cushioning, or lean against a wall for back support.

2. Lower your eyelids, but don't close your eyes completely.

3. Breathe normally. Give yourself time to tune in to the rhythm of your breathing.

4. Turn your attention to the noise and distracting thoughts in your mind. Slowly refocus your attention on the sound of your breath. Give yourself a little time to tune in to the sound of your breath. Begin to experience the sensation of your breath. Concentrate on volume, pitch, and pace. Is it louder, higher, and faster when inhaling or exhaling? Begin to visualize your lungs sucking your breath in and forcing it out again. As you concentrate on your breath, have you noticed that your mind is a little quieter?

5. By now you probably are becoming distracted by random thoughts flying across the front of your brain. Thoughts happen independent of your will. This is the challenge of meditation: Let your thoughts go. Observe random thoughts with detachment. Do not react and do not grab hold. Let your thoughts wash over you like a wave. Chant silently "let go," and refocus your attention on the sound of your breath.

6. After meditating for three to five minutes, think and write about the experience. Was it hard to concentrate? Did it get any easier? What thoughts surfaced? How did you react to them? What do you think caused you to react in this way? Is there an emotion attached to your reaction, like fear, frustration, or anxiety? Do you observe a repeated or habitual behavior in your reaction, like negative self-talk or giving up?

As with most things in yoga, meditation is about the journey rather than the destination. Meditation will become more satisfying over time if you practice regularly. Start with short, three-minute or five-minute meditation practices a few times a week. Let your biorhythms guide you in choosing the time of day to meditate. Some people enjoy morning meditation; others are more alert in the afternoon.

Like yoga practice, every meditation practice will be different. Some days your mind will slip easily into the meditation flow. Other days your mind will be battling the undertow of the day's distractions. This is a natural part of the meditation experience. Your reactions to the experience are what count. Do you allow frustrations to overwhelm you or do you persist in your meditation? Use your journal to record the insights you learn during meditation.

Just remember: It's meditation practice, not meditation perfect.

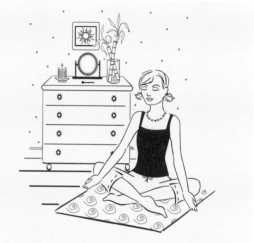

CREATING A SANCTUARY

Every girl needs a space of her own, a place where she can tune out the world and tune in to herself. Many cultures feature the tradition of a retreat for self-reflection. In the privacy of your own company, you can finally hear yourself think, put your thoughts in order, and make sense of your world.

Visit your private space to practice yoga, meditate, write in your journal, think inspiring thoughts, or just lie back and let your imagination wander and see where it lands.

With a little creativity, almost any corner can be made into a private sanctuary. For ideas on how to organize your space for maximum inspiration, look to the East. In Feng Shui, the Chinese art of placement, rooms and household objects are organized to restore balance and harmony in the home. Vastu is the Indian system of designing your space to promote inner peace.

To create a personal retreat, all you need is a small space or place that you can claim as your own. Give your retreat a name and use your yoga mat to define its boundaries. Make entering and leaving your sanctuary a ritual by ringing a chime or bell.

Surround yourself with objects that reflect your personality. Cultivate a nature preserve with plants and flowers. They will refresh the air and add color to your space. Create an Indian temple with candles, incense, and a fat Buddha. If art stimulates your imagination, hang posters nearby. Soothing music, from the classical canon to rhythmic percussion produced by modern musicians, provides the soundtrack to your voyage. (See page 101 for music recommendations.)

DOG AND CAT POSE

Start on your hands and knees. Place your hands firmly on the floor directly below your shoulders, arms straight.

Inhale: Lift your tailbone and your chin and chest, bending your head back. You will be stretching your neck and lowering your back as deeply as you can.

Exhale: Carefully tuck your chin to your chest—you will be gently stretching your neck in the opposite direction as you contract your abdominal muscles and round your back. Use your breath to create a comfortable rhythm to loosen your spine from your neck all the way to your lower back.

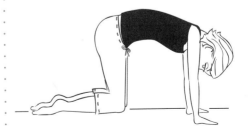

Repeat this sequence five or six times.

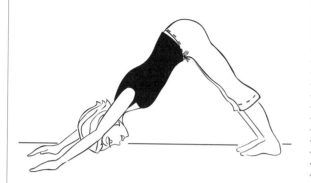

DOWN DOG

Start on your hands and knees, arms shoulder-width apart, palms pressed into the floor. Do not lock your elbows.

Inhale: Standing on the balls of your feet, lift your hips toward the ceiling and straighten your arms and legs. Tuck your chin and look back toward your belly button.

Exhale: Start to push your heels toward the floor. Continue to push your palms into the floor for stability, but let your legs do most of the work of holding you up. Continue pressing both heels toward the floor. Stay in this pose for a few breaths.

STANDING KNEE SQUEEZE

Stand tall and steady, hands on hips. Shift your weight to your right leg and press your right foot firmly into the floor for balance.

Inhale: Bend your left knee and raise it to hip height. Using one or both hands, hug your knee as close to your body as you can. Take a few breaths here.

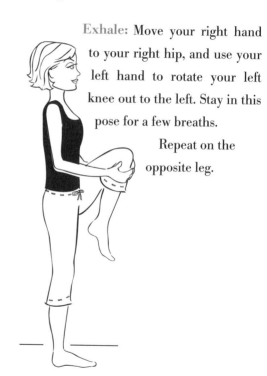

Exhale: Move your right hand to your right hip, and use your left hand to rotate your left knee out to the left. Stay in this pose for a few breaths.

Repeat on the opposite leg.

EAGLE

From a standing position, shift your weight to your right leg and bend your knee slightly. Touch your left foot to the floor for balance. Cross your left leg over your right leg at the knee. If you can, hook your left foot behind the calf of your right leg. Both of your knees are bent in this pose. Cross your left arm over your right arm at the elbow, then twist your forearms toward your body until your palms face each other. Touch your palms if you can.

Exhale: Bend your knees a little deeper. Round your upper back and stretch your arms by pushing your elbows forward and away from your body. You should feel a gentle stretch in your shoulders. Remain in this pose for three to five breaths.

Repeat on the opposite side.

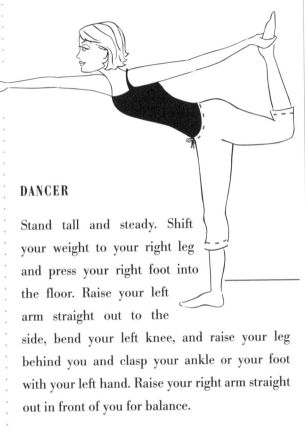

DANCER

Stand tall and steady. Shift your weight to your right leg and press your right foot into the floor. Raise your left arm straight out to the side, bend your left knee, and raise your leg behind you and clasp your ankle or your foot with your left hand. Raise your right arm straight out in front of you for balance.

Inhale: Slowly and gently, push your left foot into your left hand and bend forward from your waist a few inches.

Exhale: Raise your chin and arch your back slightly. Hold this pose for a few breaths.

Repeat on the opposite leg.

Chronic stress and poor nutrition often go hand in hand. Stress can create the impulse to overeat or to skip meals. These muffins are loaded with fiber, and the fresh carrots provide complex carbohydrates that stimulate the production of serotonin, the brain's natural tranquilizer.

YOGA CHICK'S CARROT CAKE MUFFINS

1 cup low-fat plain yogurt

⅓ cup applesauce

½ teaspoon vanilla

2 tablespoons milk

1 egg

2 cups whole wheat flour

⅓ cup sugar

3 teaspoons baking powder

1 teaspoon cinnamon

dash of salt

1 cup shredded carrots

Optional: ½ cup raisins or dried cranberries and/or ½ cup walnuts

Preheat oven to 400 degrees F. Line six regular-size muffin tins with paper baking cups.

Beat the yogurt, applesauce, vanilla, milk, and egg in a large bowl until well mixed.

Stir in flour, sugar, baking powder, cinnamon, and salt, and mix gently. The batter will be a little lumpy.

Stir in carrots, and raisins and nuts if you wish to include them.

Spoon into baking cups, dividing the batter evenly.

Bake 20–25 minutes or until golden brown. Remove muffins from the baking tin and cool on a wire rack.

Note: Would you like muffins for breakfast but feel too rushed in the morning to make them? Prepare the batter ahead of time, pour it into the lined muffin tins, and seal the tins in a freezer bag. When you're ready to enjoy them, take them out of the bag and bake the frozen muffins in a 400-degree oven for about 30 minutes or until golden brown.

BOAT

Lie on your stomach with your forehead touching the floor. Clasp your hands behind your back.

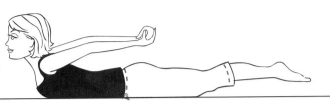

Inhale: Raise your head, neck, shoulders, and chest from the floor.

Exhale: Release.

Inhale: Raise your head, neck, shoulders, chest, and legs from the floor.

Exhale: Release.
Repeat three times.

SEATED FORWARD FOLD

Sit on the floor comfortably with your legs extended straight in front of you.

Inhale: Lift your arms overhead.

Exhale: Gently bend forward from the waist and touch or clasp your feet. Stay in this position for a few breaths. On each exhalation, extend your reach a little farther.

BRIDGE

Lie on your back, legs hip-width apart and knees bent, arms parallel to your body, fingers pointing toward your feet.

Inhale: Contract your quadriceps, glutes, and abdomen to raise your hips from the floor.

Variation: Place your hands at your lower back for more support. Stay in this pose for three breaths.
Repeat three times.

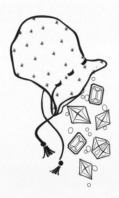

ROCK STARS

At the center of some of mankind's oldest legends are stories about the mysterious powers of precious and semiprecious gems. These rock stars generate unique vibrational energy that can create good luck and good health. The most fun—and fashionable—way to tap into the healing powers of gems is to wear them as jewelry. A wide variety of affordable stones are available in jewelry stores, boutiques, and specialty stores that carry crystals. Jewelry—earrings, wrist and ankle bracelets, and necklaces—does double duty as an accessory on and off your mat. Choose the gem that will most enhance your yoga or meditation practice. Just remember to remove dangly pieces before practice.

Moonstone. In love? A soft, ivory stone that looks like moonlight on a cloudy night, moonstone can attract good luck in a budding romance or protect an existing relationship.

Topaz. Shooting for a promotion? Yellow topaz promotes a good public reputation and prestige in career or business ventures.

Peridot. Owe someone an apology? Citrus-green peridot increases integrity and nurtures humility.

Cat's-eye. Who couldn't use nine lives? The polished brown or yellow stone features a vertical streak that looks like the eye of a cat. Wear cat's-eye for strength and cunning.

Tourmaline. Does your piggy bank need fattening up? This multicolored gem brings wealth. Store it with your savings and see if your money grows.

Amber. Staring in the face of a deadline? Wear amber to stimulate your creativity and intellect.

Aquamarine. Need to see into the future? To

develop stronger intuition and psychic gifts, wear aquamarine.

Lapis lazuli. Going into battle on the soccer field? The gem of the warrior, a lapis lazuli will shore up your courage and protect you from enemies.

Rose quartz. Communication breakdown? The romantic pink rose quartz promotes trust in relationships and creates clarity that helps you see the other person's point of view.

Crystals. Could you use extra protection? Worn as dagger-shaped pendants, crystals are known for their healing powers.

SHOULDER STAND

Lie on the floor, legs close together.

Inhale: Bend your knees and roll your hips up from the floor. Place your hands on your lower back for support and continue to roll back until you are lying on your upper back and shoulders. Flex your feet and extend your legs straight up. Remain in this pose for three to five breaths.

CHILD'S POSE

Kneel on the floor with your feet together and your knees wide apart. Sit back on your heels. Bend forward from your waist over your knees. Place your forehead on the floor. Relax your shoulders and let your arms fall comfortably to the floor at your sides.

PEACEFUL POSE

Lie flat on your back on the floor with your arms and legs open a comfortable distance apart, but no more than a few inches. Breathe naturally.

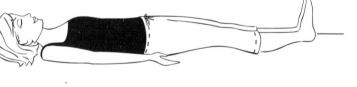

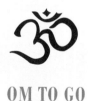

OM TO GO

Just when the caterpillar thought her life was over,

she became a butterfly.

CHAPTER EIGHT

Even Yoga Chicks Get the Blues

Use yoga to soothe your spirits.

veryone feels a little melancholy from time to time. A blue mood is usually caused by something you can put your finger on, like a disappointing phone call or the premenstrual blahs. But sometimes blue moods come, well, from out of the blue. A change in the weather or a sad song on the radio may be all it takes to dampen your spirits.

If a blue cloud settles over you, treat yourself with the same compassion you would show a friend. Your feelings are important and acknowledging them is the first step toward soothing them. Usually your lousy mood is trying to tell you something, and your yoga mat is a safe place to sit quietly and listen to what it has to say.

Change is a major source of the blues. Letting go of something, like a friend, disrupts your sense of your world and can make you feel insecure. This yoga practice will help you manage a blue mood by finding the balance between continuity and change. The back bends in this practice increase in difficulty with each pose. Pause and take a look at how you react during the transitions. Pay attention to how you adapt to the increasing effort that's required with each new pose.

A strong back projects self-confidence, integrity, and character. More important, back bends expose your chest and heart, which can help you get comfortable with feeling vulnerable. Back bends remind us that happiness begins in the heart and that love begins with loving ourselves.

When the blues set in, many yoginis look to the lotus flower for perspective. Every day, the lotus flower pushes through muddy waters to blossom pure and clean in the sun. The daily journey of the lotus flower reminds us that tomorrow always comes, the sun will shine again, and your spirits will return to normal.

Scent is another one of nature's most powerful mood boosters. Learn more about how to apply the principles of aromatherapy to boost your spirits.

One final thought before you start your practice: If your blue mood persists for more than a day or two, please talk to a trusted friend, your family, or a doctor. It could be a symptom of a more serious problem like depression, which is a biological problem that can be treated. And remember, even poor eating and sleeping habits or a change in the weather can have a powerful effect on your mood.

Practice tip: Use your breath to guide you gently into the back bends in this sequence. Use each inhalation to expand and each exhalation to release a little deeper. Just like in life, sometimes the most subtle movement generates the biggest benefit, so don't overdo it.

MOUNTAIN POSE

Stand tall with your feet hip-width apart, chest lifted, arms at your sides with the palms facing your body. Distribute your weight evenly over both feet, tuck your tailbone, and contract your abdomen. Feel yourself becoming strong and stable, standing on your own two feet.

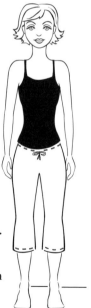

Inhale: Start Victory Breathing. Once you feel centered and connected to your breath, begin your yoga practice.

STANDING ARM RAISE

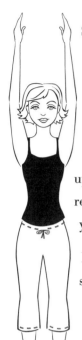

Inhale: Reach out from your shoulders, raise your arms out to the sides of your body and reach up over your head, fingertips touching. Raise your chin to look up at your hands and continue to reach toward the ceiling, feeling your spine lengthen.

Exhale: Lower your arms and straighten your head and back.

STANDING FORWARD FOLD, ARMS FOLDED

Inhale: Raise your arms out to the sides of your body and reach up over your head. Raise your chin to look up at your hands and continue to reach toward the ceiling, feeling your spine lengthen.

Exhale: Tuck your chin to your chest, bend forward from your waist, arms out to the side, palms facing down. Fold your arms one over the other, clasping your elbows. Bend your knees and point the crown of your head toward the floor. Feel your lower back stretch. Stay in this position for a few breaths.

UNDULATING BACK

Inhale: Slowly rise one vertebra at a time, arms and head hanging limp, until you are standing tall.

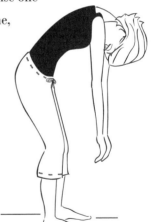

CRESCENT MOON

Inhale: Raise your arms out to the sides of your body and reach up over your head, fingertips touching.

Exhale: Stretch up and over to your right, feeling the stretch on the entire right side of your body. Hold this pose for a few breaths. Repeat on the opposite side.

STANDING CAMEL

Inhale: Place the heels of both hands at the small of your back, fingers pointing down. Roll your shoulders back and lift your chest.

Exhale: Carefully lean back into a gentle back bend.

HALF COBRA

Lie down on your stomach and prop yourself up on your forearms, hands placed directly below your shoulders.

Inhale: Resting on your forearms, use your shoulders and upper back muscles to lift your head, neck, and shoulders from the floor. Look straight ahead. Hold this pose for three to five breaths.

FULL COBRA

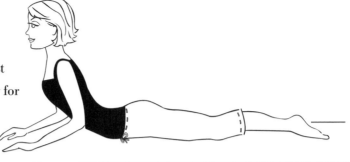

Inhale: Use your upper back muscles to lift your head, neck, shoulders, and chest from the floor, using your forearms only for support. Look straight ahead. Hold this pose for three to five breaths.

Wise women who were knowledgeable about the healing power of herbs held high positions in ancient societies. Their herbal remedies kept tribal hunters strong and treated diseases.

Today a renewed interest in herbal medicine is under way as people seek natural, more gentle remedies. High-quality herbal tea is one of the most accessible ways to take your herbal medicine. Most grocery stores offer a variety of prepackaged herbal tea and most health food stores offer a wide variety of dried herbs with which you can make your own combinations.

Chamomile contains calming essential oils that promote sleep and soothe stomach upsets. Make a cup of chamomile tea a bedtime ritual and soon you will be enjoying sweet dreams!

CALMING HERBAL TEA

In a teapot or saucepan, combine:

1 teaspoon dried chamomile

1 teaspoon dried lemongrass

½ teaspoon dried mint

1 whole clove

1 cup boiling water

Steep for five minutes. Strain the tea through a tea strainer. Add a bit of table sugar, stevia, or Splenda to taste.

Makes 1 serving.

SUPPORTED SEATED FORWARD FOLD

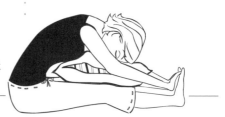

Sit on the floor with your legs extended straight in front of you.

Place a pillow on your thighs.

Inhale: Lift your arms overhead.

Exhale: Gently bend forward from the waist, reaching toward your feet and resting your head and chest on the pillow. Stay in this position for a few breaths.

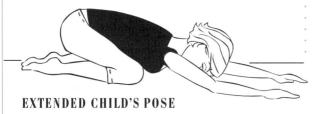

EXTENDED CHILD'S POSE

Kneel on the floor with your feet together and your knees wide apart. Sit back on your heels. Bend forward from your waist over your knees. Place your forehead on the floor. Try to lower your buttocks to your heels. Extend your arms straight out in front of you, palms flat on the floor.

SUPPORTED PEACEFUL POSE

Lie flat on your back on the floor with your arms and legs open a comfortable distance apart, but no more than a few inches. Prop your knees up with a rolled blanket, pillow or cushion. You might also like to use a lavender-scented eye pillow. Cover yourself with a blanket to stay warm.

Breathe naturally. Beginning with your feet, let go, totally relaxing. Try not to think, just enjoy the feeling of sinking into the floor. Stay in this position as long as you like—but don't fall asleep!

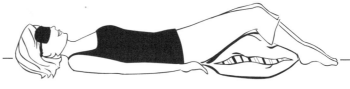

FEET UP THE WALL

An alternative to Peaceful Pose is to lie on your back with your legs propped up against a wall. Stay in this position as long as you are comfortable.

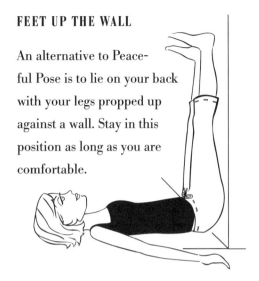

HAPPINESS FROM THE INSIDE OUT

Happy people radiate a glow that inspires others to feel good, too. People who say they are happy have fewer illnesses, experience more satisfying relationships, and generally perform better in school and in their jobs. Study after study shows that money, prestige, and status do not create happiness. So what makes them so darned happy?

Truly happy people have three things in common: perspective about their own life, the feeling that they can make changes when necessary, and the practice of acceptance. They are also realistic about happiness. Some people experience highs and then fall into a funk when life returns to normal, whereas happy people accept the fact that life is full of ups and downs. Happy people look for satisfaction every day in meaningful work and close relationships.

Put It into Perspective

- "This too shall pass" means that everything changes and your current situation will also change. What is important today may not be as important tomorrow, or next week or next year.
- Sometimes all we need is the smallest shift in perspective to see things in a different light. Viewing a challenge as an opportunity to stretch yourself changes your approach to tough tasks and helps you to grow and mature.
- Be happy today. Appreciate what is going on in your life right now. Enduring happiness is taking

pleasure from life's common events. Let flowers delight you with their color and smell. Look to the stars and let them wow you. Rent your favorite movie, watch it with a friend, and share a good laugh or a good cry. Or both!

Change What Can Be Changed

- Change your self-talk. Is your inner voice sabotaging you with negative thinking? Look at yourself in the mirror and start talking to your best friend.
- Change your attitude. It may sound like a cliché, but it bears repeating: Look at a glass as half full rather than half empty.
- Put on a happy face. Even happy people experience an occasional down mood, but they have mastered acting happy by continuing to smile and projecting a positive attitude. Other people respond positively to happy, confident people, which is enough to make you feel happier.

Let It Go

- Accept yourself. We all make mistakes and do or say things we later wish we could do over.

Happy people don't flog themselves for making mistakes. They examine their behavior, vow to learn from it, forgive themselves, and move on with self-respect.

- Let go. It is human nature to form attachments to people, places, ideas, and things. However, though it takes time, it's possible to hang on to the feeling of love but to let go of the attachment. Only when you let go can you truly be happy.

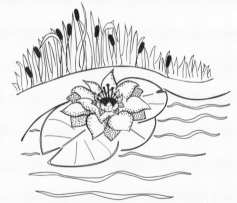

THE FLOWER OF LIGHT: THE SYMBOLIC LOTUS

For thousands of years, in cultures that practice yoga the lotus flower has appeared as the symbol of creation, purity, and enlightenment. In Hindu mythology, the lotus flower is symbolic of the goddess Lakshmi, wife of the Hindu god Vishnu. Lakshmi is shown in Hindu art seated on her lotus blossom throne, representing the mother of creation and feminine beauty. The legends about Buddha present him seated on a lotus blossom at the time of his spiritual enlightenment. The violet lotus blossom at the crown chakra represents spiritual flowering and wisdom.

Lush with petals, lotus flowers grow in shallow ponds and muddy rivers surrounded by lily pads, clusters of its large, waxy leaves that float on top of the water. These mysterious flowers open and close with the cycle of the sun. At night, the blossoms close and retreat below the surface of the water. Each morning, the pointed tip of the flower breaks the muddy surface of the water and opens its face to the sun as a pristine blossom.

The lotus is a metaphor for our own lives. With our feet grounded solidly, we face each day unfolding as beautiful pure flower blossoms, reaching for the light that will nurture our spirits.

SOOTHE YOUR SPIRITS THROUGH SCENT

Have you ever wondered why a favorite smell, like the scent of baking bread or fresh-cut grass, gives you a big smile? Of all the five human senses, smell has the most immediate effect on our mood.

Aromatherapy is a nature's way of enhancing our feelings of well-being.

It works by tapping into our powerful sense of smell through the pleasant aromas of flowers and plants. The right scent can inspire you during a long evening at work, calm your rattled nerves before a big presentation, or lift your flagging spirits after a disappointment.

Essential Oils

The ancient Egyptians were the first to extract essential oils, highly concentrated essences, from flowers and plants. They believed that the aroma of the plant or flower carried its life force, which stimulates natural healing in humans. The character of each essential oil is identified by its source: floral, fruit, herb, leaf, wood, spice, seed, root, or resin. Some essential oils express a combination of characters. Today, high-quality essential oils are available in many health food stores and pharmacies. They are packaged in small, dark glass to protect their delicate essences from sunlight. A drop or two of essential oil warmed in a diffuser carries a lovely fragrance into the room.

Essential oils are versatile and easy to use. Create your own signature products by scenting your laundry detergent, bathwater, shower soap, and body lotion with an essential oil. Be careful, though, because some essential oils are powerful and can irritate your skin if you use too much. Read the instructions that come with your oil to learn how to use it safely.

Incense

Incense was known throughout the ancient world, though it was the Chinese who perfected incense sticks. An incense stick is formed from the ground essences of flowers and plants that are then com-

pressed into a slender stick. When the stick is lit, ribbons of slender smoke unfurl a beautiful fragrance. Incense comes in cones as well as sticks, and is burned in a small holder. High-quality incense is widely available in the same types of stores that carry essential oils.

Candles

Scented candles are a safe and convenient way to get a small dose of aromatherapy when you need it. Choose your candles wisely. Some candles are heavily perfumed rather than scented with essential oils. Soy-based candles are environmentally friendly and do not leave a smoky residue on the walls.

What's Your Scent?

These scent personality types have been adapted from the book *The Fragrant Mind,* by Valerie Ann Wormwood, one of the world's foremost experts in aromatherapy. Choose the scent that most closely matches your personality.

Romantic: If you are joyful, creative, and feminine, then call yourself a romantic. Everyone loves your charming, innocent nature. Fill your essential oil cabinet with classic florals like jasmine, rose, and tuberose.

A Friend Indeed: People admire you as a good friend. You are loyal and sport a drip-dry shoulder for friends to cry on. Fill your essential oil cabinet with the citrus fruit scents—lemon, lime, orange, and grapefruit.

Natural Nurturer: If your home-baked brownies are legend, you could be a generous and affectionate earth mother. Fill your essential oil cabinet with herbal essences like basil, mint, and sage.

Live Wire: Your motto is "Work hard, play hard." Adults are impressed with your intelligence and ambition, but your friends know you as the party girl who lights up the room with your sparkling personality. Fill your essential oil cabinet with spicy ginger, cinnamon, and clove.

The Activist: You are courageous and want to change the world. You split your time between animal rights, environmental protection, and the Vegan Gourmet Club. Fill your essential oil cabinet with strong woods like cedar, pine, and sandalwood.

Fine-Tune Your Moods with Aromatherapy

The "Aromatherapy Rx" chart identifies the characteristics of some of the most common essential oils. You can use that or some of the following ideas to get you started on creating your own aromatherapy rituals.

De-stress and rest. When your stress meter reaches the red zone, calm down in a soothing bath scented with lavender, eucalyptus, or chamomile.

During the day, carry a plastic bag that contains a tissue, a handkerchief, or cotton balls scented with a few drops of lavender or eucalyptus. Take a whiff from your bag from time to time during the day.

Stimulate your energy. Wake up your senses after a day in school or at work. Light a candle or a stick of incense or burn a drop of oil in a diffuser, using one of these scents: cinnamon, ginger, or mint. Any time you need a pick-me-up, try a quick shower and lather up with grapefruit- or lime-scented shower soap.

Cultivate peacefulness and well-being. To create a comfy mood at a gathering of friends, burn a drop or two of sandalwood oil. New cute guy coming over to hang out and watch a movie? Set the mood with patchouli.

AROMATHERAPY RX

Essential Oil	Character	Emotional Response
Chamomile	Harmonizing	Relaxation
Jasmine	Sensual	Sensitivity
Lavender	Calming	Harmony
Rose	Loving	Joy
Tuberose	Spontaneous	Self-expression
Ylang-Ylang	Unifying	Self-confidence
Grapefruit	Cheerful	Happiness
Lemon	Purifying	Clarity
Basil	Stimulating	Concentration
Mint	Awakening	Refreshment
Rosemary	Strengthening	Confidence
Cinnamon	Warming	Invigoration
Eucalyptus	Balanced	Centeredness
Patchouli	Grounded	Balance
Ginger	Encouraging	Courage
Vetiver	Wise	Integrity
Coriander	Motivating	Optimism
Sandalwood	Enlightening	Serenity

OM TO GO

To change our lives,

we must first change our minds.

CHAPTER NINE

Two Oms Are Better Than One

Nourish your relationships.

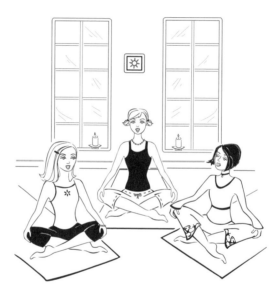

Yoga is more fun with friends! Relationships give meaning and purpose to our lives, and sharing a yoga practice is a fun way to nourish important relationships and relate to your friends.

Yoga practice is a great way to spend quality time with someone special because it can build a bridge to better communication. Yoga works to break through barriers, like lack of self-confidence or the ability to trust other people, that prevent us from communicating from our hearts. After practice, you may feel more open and less defensive and able to talk more honestly about your feelings and what's going on in your life.

The poses in this chapter promote union and understanding between partners. Practicing with a partner requires verbal and nonverbal communication, which will reward you with a new understanding of your friend.

Dancing is another way to access your intuition and cultivate a higher consciousness. Yoga trance dancing is an energetic, free-form body and breath extravaganza. The rhythmic music and pounding percussion of these music selections will unleash your creative energy. Don't be shy—yoga is not about how you look, it's about how you feel. Wind down from trance dancing with life-affirming music that will restore calm to your gathering. If you choose to apply henna tattoos together, that sense of calmness will give you the steady hand you'll need.

Many yoga principles have been influenced by Buddha, the rebel who launched a religion based on meditation. The great lesson Buddha left to the world is that wisdom and compassion are our greatest virtues.

THE ART OF THE HENNA TATTOO

Adorning your body with exotic tattoos using henna, an all-natural, temporary dye, is not only a means of artistic expression, but it can attract romantic love and prosperity, too! Called *mehndi,* henna art is used to elaborately decorate the hands and feet of brides in India, North Africa, and the Middle East. Mehndi art is also used for everyday adornment by the rest of us, and can be viewed as a fashion statement, an expression of femininity and sexuality, or an exotic form of transformation and transcendence.

Designs range from detailed flowers, constellations, and paisley patterns to bold geometric shapes. Besides decorating your hands and feet, try a henna sunburst around your belly button or a big henna flower on your shoulder with vines creeping down your back. Henna is generally a reddish brown, but can be tinted in vivid colors to enhance its beauty. Henna tattoo kits are widely available, easy to use, and a lot of fun—especially with friends. Check your local beauty salon, too. Many salons now offer henna tattoos. If you're in a beach community, stroll the boardwalk and you are likely to find a henna artist just waiting to adorn you with her most beautiful work. Make henna tattoos your own individual expression of Yoga Chick style.

Partner poses help you develop keen perception about other people. Your partner's breathing and pace will tell you a lot about them. If your partner is rushed or seems a little nervous, you can help her calm down by breathing more deeply yourself.

PARTNERS BREATHING

Sit in a comfortable cross-legged position facing each other. Appoint a leader to begin the chant. Inhale deeply and chant "Ohhhhmmm" slowly until you are out of breath. Feel the vibrations in the back of your throat. Repeat three times.

Sit back to back in a comfortable cross-legged position. Your hands may be folded in your lap or poised on your knees, palms facing up. Begin to synchronize your breathing, paying close attention to your own breath and your partner's rhythms. Stay in this pose for a few minutes.

PARTNERS TWIST

Remain seated back to back with your partner. Extend your arms out to your sides, parallel with the floor, and clasp wrists. Synchronize your inhalation and slowly twist to the right. Synchronize your exhalation and slowly twist to the left. Repeat this sequence three times.

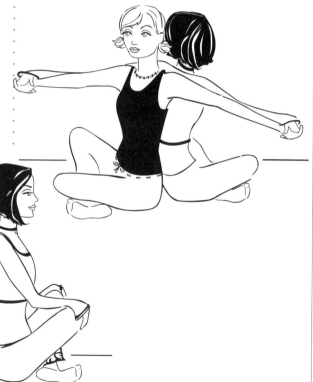

PARTNERS CHILD'S POSE

One partner should kneel on the floor, feet together and knees wide apart, bent forward from the waist, forehead touching the floor. Shoulders should be relaxed and arms comfortably extended forward or draped along the side of the body.

The second partner should lie back over her partner, heads pointing the same direction, to achieve a back bend. Adjust yourselves until you feel comfortable, with no strain on either partner's neck or lower back. Hold this pose for three to five breaths.

Change positions and repeat.

TUNE IN WITH YOGA MUSIC

Before, during, or after—music is a great way to enhance your yoga practice.

Warm up with *Yoga Trance Dance* by Shiva Rea, an inspirational yogini who has brought modern music to an ancient and primal art. Madonna's yoga-themed *Ray of Light* will inspire your imagination with its global music beat. For something totally different, try *Gus Gus vs. T-World* by Gus Gus, an electronic artist with an energetic rhythm.

On a softer note, appropriate for yoga practice or winding down afterwards, play *Acoustic Soul* by India Arie, *Truth* by Mantra Girl, *Buddha Lounge* and *Buddha Lounge 2* by various artists, *Classical Music for Yoga* by Peter Davison, *Surfacing* by Sarah McLachlan, *Songbird* by Eva Cassidy, *Parachutes* by Coldplay, and anything by the artist Enya.

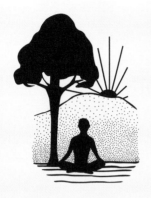

WIDE AWAKE:
BUDDHISM FOR BEGINNERS

What is Buddhism?

Buddhism is a religion practiced by more than 300 million people around the world. The word *Buddha* means "awakened one." Buddhists seek enlightenment, or spiritual awakening, as their goal. They believe that leading a moral life and living with awareness and mindfulness of one's desires and actions will result in wisdom and understanding.

Who was Buddha?

Siddhartha Gautama, a wealthy young prince from Nepal, knew that wealth and social prestige did not promise happiness. He left his family and spent many years in extreme conditions pursuing enlightenment. After a long night spent meditating under the broad canopy of an old bodhi tree, Siddhartha found the answer to human suffering and declared himself enlightened. He became Buddha, or "the awakened one," and established a new religion based on his teachings.

What did Buddha discover?

He realized that the source of all human suffering is desire. Put another way, seeing what we want to see rather than seeing reality causes suffering. Buddhism is the philosophy of acceptance. Buddha spent the rest of his long life teaching people how to avoid suffering and be truly happy. He developed these principles in the Four Noble Truths and the Eightfold Path.

What are Buddhist virtues?

The Four Noble Truths lay out the framework for the human condition.

- *First Noble Truth:* Suffering is an inescapable part of life, and we all suffer fear and pain to some extent.

- *Second Noble Truth:* Suffering is caused by desire and expectation. For every desire that is satisfied, a new one rises to replace it.
- *Third Noble Truth:* By detaching ourselves from desire, we learn to live in the moment and appreciate the gifts of the present. The past is gone; the future is yet to be lived. True happiness is in enjoying the here and now.
- *Fourth Noble Truth:* Following the Eightfold Path leads to the end of suffering. This is the guidebook for moral living that leads to wisdom.

What does Buddhism mean by "wisdom"?

Developing wisdom by cultivating compassion and loving-kindness is a central virtue in Buddhism. These virtues combine the heart and the intellectual mind. Buddhism asks you to take responsibility for what you believe by listening to other points of view with an open mind and open heart, examining facts objectively, and courageously changing your beliefs after careful analysis. True wisdom comes from thinking for yourself by using your head for analysis and your heart for empathy with the human condition.

In Buddhism, compassion is defined literally as the wish that all sentient beings be free of suffering. Compassion is the emotional side of our nature. It is empathizing with the feelings of other people. Buddhism also promotes compassion for oneself. Developing self-love and self-respect is the first step in developing compassion for other people.

What is loving-kindness?

Buddhism believes that by changing your thoughts, you change your life. The practice of loving-kindness replaces negative thoughts and actions with compassionate, loving thoughts and actions. It is the Buddhist version of the power of positive thinking, without the sentimentality. Loving-kindness is about accepting people and circumstances as they are. Like compassion, loving-kindness begins with an acceptance of yourself, with all your faults and virtues. Loving-kindness does not mean playing the pushover to people who are mean or destructive toward you. It simply helps condition you to not respond with anger and hostility toward negative people. By practicing loving-kindness, you forgive others their faults and move on, detaching yourself from the negative emotion of the situation.

What is karma?

Karma is the spiritual law of cause and effect. It means we do not act in a vacuum, but that our actions have consequences. The energy we project will come back to us in the form of a reaction, either in this life or the next. Recognizing this law encourages us to take responsibility for our actions and to live by the moral laws of Buddhism.

Why do Buddhists meditate?

Buddhism emphasizes the powers of observation. Through meditation you practice self-observation. There are many types of meditation practices that focus on emotions, feelings, thoughts, physical sensations. With the self-awareness that you cultivate through meditation, it is possible to see yourself more clearly and to change, evolve, and adapt in ways that promote happiness and equanimity.

What is mindfulness?

Mindfulness is the ability to concentrate fully on the present and to resist distractions. We all too often rush through our busy lives paying only partial attention to the food we eat, the things we say to people, and our actions. Buddhism teaches us to be mindful in all our actions and interactions as a way to fully participate in the present moment.

How do I learn more about Buddhism?

Often yoginis enjoy Buddhism and find it compatible with their yoga practice and healthy, natural lifestyle. It's possible to explore the philosophy of Buddhism without converting to the religion. His Holiness the Dalai Lama is the foremost spiritual leader in the Buddhist world today. He has written many books about Buddhism and Buddhist principles that are enjoyed by people of all religions around the world.

OM TO GO

Dance like no one is watching; sing as if no one can hear. Live life to its fullest!

PART III

Yoga Chick's Next Steps

CHAPTER 10

Choosing a Yoga Style

You can find a yoga class just about anywhere: health clubs, community centers, hospitals and health care facilities, and schools, as well as yoga studios. Over the last decade many styles of yoga have emerged, and it can be confusing to choose the right class for you. The good news is that each style focuses on the same core principle: using your breath to unite your mind, body, and spirit!

Hatha Yoga

This term is used generically in the West to refer to a gentle yoga class.

Vinyasa-Style Yoga, Also Called Flow Yoga

Vinyasa uses breathing to link a series of poses in a dancelike flow. Yoga studios offer classes by level of experience.

Level I classes are for beginning yoga students who are taught yoga breathing, along with sitting, standing, and other basic yoga poses.

Level II classes are for students who are comfortable performing basic poses at a faster pace. In Level II classes, students learn advanced variations of basic yoga poses and inversions. Inversions are upside-down yoga poses like Headstand and Handstand.

Level III classes are for advanced yoga students. In Level III classes, students should be able to perform a basic inversion pose without assistance from the teacher.

Ashtanga Yoga

Sometimes called power yoga, Ashtanga yoga is a popular, fast-paced and demanding style. The Ashtanga school of yoga features six separate practices, each progressively more difficult, that are designed to generate heat and energy. If you have been practicing Flow yoga and are comfortable performing basic yoga poses, give an Ashtanga Primary Series class a try.

Iyengar Yoga

Also sometimes called gentle yoga, Iyengar yoga was developed by B. K. S. Iyengar and focuses on the precise alignment of each pose. The Iyengar style of yoga is a great way to learn the basic poses correctly. Each pose may use props, including belts, chairs, blocks, and blankets. You will not work up a sweat in an Iyengar class, but you will learn the basics in a safe environment.

Viniyoga

Viniyoga was developed by T. K. V. Desikachar, the son of Krishnamacharya. The poses are performed like Flow yoga, but the teacher's dialogue promotes personal transformation through the practice.

Bikram Yoga

If you like it hot, you may want to try Bikram yoga, a sequence of twenty-six traditional yoga poses performed in a studio that is heated like a sauna. The minimum temperature in a Bikram studio is 105 degrees. Only studios formally affiliated with the Bikram College of Yoga India may call themselves Bikram Yoga. You may see "hot yoga" offered at a studio or health club, but it will not be the same practice.

Kundalini

If you like your yoga on the exotic side, try Kundalini, an ancient and esoteric school. It combines yoga poses, vigorous breathing, and chanting to awaken the energy coiled at the base of the spine.

Anusara

Anusara means "flowing with grace." It is a vigorous and inspirational yoga practice in the Vinyasa-Flow style. Anusara combines the discipline of Iyengar yoga with the spirituality of Kundalini yoga.

Sample several yoga styles to find a practice you like. Also try different teachers. Yoga teachers bring their personal style and spirit to class, so one teacher may inspire you more or less than another. You can expect every yoga teacher to care about your comfort, safety, and spirit in class.

Taking a Class

Reading this book is a great way to start a yoga practice and develop good habits. It may fulfill all need for yoga. At some point, though, you may want to take a yoga class. Yoga teachers are trained to help you perform every pose, even the most basic poses, safely and comfortably. Once you have mastered basic yoga poses, a good teacher can help you advance to more challenging poses.

Look for a reputable yoga studio in your community. If you're a teen, look for classes offered specifically for teens. Otherwise, start out with a beginner's class.

Yoga studios range from simple rooms with hardwood floors to more elaborate spaces decorated with exotic fabric wall coverings and art. Almost all yoga studios burn incense. Sometimes new smells can give you a headache, but most of the time the smell of incense burning is pleasant and creates a calm, peaceful environment.

You may take your own mat to yoga class, but most studios provide mats, blocks, blankets, and other props. Arrive at the studio dressed in your yoga clothes, but carry street clothes to change into after class.

Behave courteously toward others and you will fit in fine. Be prepared to remove your street shoes as soon as you enter a studio. Yoga studios are quiet. People are meditating and preparing for practice. Quietly enter the studio, then pause to survey the room and choose a place that looks comfortable to you. Perhaps you like practicing near a window. If it's your first yoga class in a studio, you may want to take a place near the teacher. Claim your space by unfolding your mat and settle in comfortably. Close your eyes, concentrate on your breathing, and wait for the teacher's instructions.

Before class starts, introduce yourself to the teacher and explain that this is your first yoga class in a studio. The teacher may give you specific instructions. If you feel fatigued, unsteady, or in any way uncomfortable during yoga class, drop into Peaceful Pose, a common resting pose.

Once class begins, remember, it's your yoga practice and the only person who matters is you! If you lose your place in the sequence or don't understand the instructions, look at the teacher for guidance. If you need help, just ask the teacher. Every student in yoga class is trying to concentrate on their practice, as you should, too. Your friends will understand if you avoid giggles and chatter during yoga class. Your maturity will set an example for others.

One last piece of advice: Yoga twists on empty tummies sometimes create gas. This is a common side effect of yoga and can happen to even the most adept yoginis. If you feel the urge to pass gas, quietly leave your mat and exit the studio to relieve yourself. Return to your mat quietly and resume your practice. Your courtesy will be appreciated by your fellow yoginis.

Keep Breathing

I hope by now that you are saying, "Yoga makes me feel so good—about myself!"

Our culture is just beginning to embrace the yoga philosophy that promotes natural methods for supporting physical and mental health. Living life to its fullest can be hard work! Balancing work with rest and balancing the desire to perform with self-acceptance are yoga's most important lessons.

The beauty of yoga is that something new always lies ahead. The challenge of a vigorous Sun Salutation, for example, is your chance to explore: *Who am I? Am I made of enough determination and focus to stay with my breath through sustained effort?* The strength and stability you create in each Mountain Pose help you shape who you want to be, giving you the chance to be your truest self rather than a willow in the wind who bends to the influence of other people. And every breath you take is an opportunity to renew your confidence and optimism about the future.

Yoga is as much about your life off the mat as the exercises you perform on it. *Yoga Chick* has introduced you to many techniques and strategies for taking care of yourself and attending to your own needs. You may come back to this book or parts of it over and over again. The yoga practices are classic sequences that you can adapt to your schedule and energy level. The sections about meditation and self-reflection are just starting points. If you want to continue to expand your yoga horizons, check out the resources section for other books, videos, and Web sites.

You may choose to expand your yoga practice and to learn the more advanced poses you see in books and on magazine covers. Or perhaps you will move on to deeper meditation practices. Expanding into more advanced work, however, does not necessarily increase your appreciation of the lessons that yoga has to offer.

Whether you are in Headstand or Mountain Pose, the basic principles of yoga never change: Just breathe.

Peace,
Bess

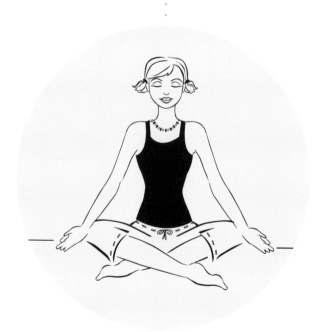

Yoga Resources

YOGA PUBLICATIONS AND WEB SITES

Yoga Journal
475 Sansome Street, Suite 850
San Francisco, CA 94111
(415) 591-0555
www.yogajournal.com

Yoga Chicago
P.O. Box 607447
Chicago, IL 60660
(773) 989-6767
www.yogachicago.com

Tricycle: The Buddhist Review
92 Vandam Street
New York, NY 10013
(212) 645-1143
www.tricycle.com

ESSENTIAL READING

Light on Yoga, by B. K. S. Iyengar. Published by Schocken Books, Allen & Unwin.

The Heart of Yoga, by T. K. V. Desikachar. Published by Inner Traditions International.

The Fragrant Mind, by Valerie Ann Wormwood. Published by New World Library.

YOGA MATS, VIDEOS, AND ACCESSORIES

Gaiam, A Lifestyle Company
360 Interlocken Boulevard
Broomfield, CO 80021
(303) 222-3600
www.gaiam.com
This online catalog company carries eco-friendly

and stylishly designed products for the mind, body, spirit, and home that support a healthy and natural lifestyle. It's a great source for yoga mats, chimes, water fountains, and other things that will enhance your private sanctuary.

HEALTH AND WELLNESS

Merz Apothecary
4716 North Lincoln Avenue
Chicago, IL 60625
(800) 252-0275
www.smallflower.com
This European-style apothecary has been in business for more than one hundred years. It carries high-quality homeopathic remedies, vitamins, supplements, and other natural medicines, as well as natural skin care, bath, aromatherapy, and other personal care products from around the world. Look for your essential oils, incense, and smudge sticks here.

The Ayurvedic Institute
11311 Menaul Boulevard N.E.
Albuquerque, NM
(505) 291-9698
www.ayurveda.com

Vegetarian Times
300 North Continental Boulevard, Suite 650
El Segundo, CA 90245
(310) 356-4100
www.vegetariantimes.com

MEDITATION RESOURCES

Meditation Station
The Meditation Society of America
P.O. Box 126
Wagontown, PA 19376
www.meditationsociety.com

The Dalai Lama Foundation
1804 Embarcadero Road, Suite 200
Palo Alto, CA 94303-3318
(650) 354-0733
www.dalailamafoundation.org
The Dalai Lama is the world's foremost Buddhist leader.

BOOKS, MUSIC, AND MEDIA

SoundsTrue
413 South Arthur Avenue
Louisville, CO 80027

(800) 333-9185

www.soundstrue.com

Sounds True offers more than five hundred titles about spiritual traditions, meditation, psychology, creativity, health and healing, self-discovery, and relationships.

Amber Lotus Publishing
5018 N.E. 22nd Avenue, Studio A
Portland, OR 97211
(877) 318-1287
www.amberlotus.com

ESPECIALLY FOR TEENAGERS

Buddha in Your Backpack: Everyday Buddhism for Teens, by Franz Metcalf. Published by Seastone Press

Just Say Om: Your Life's Journey, by Soren Gordhamer. Published by Adams Media.

Girlosophy: A Soul Survival Kit, by Anthea Paul. Published by Allen & Unwin.

YouthMoves, the Dalai Lama Foundation
1804 Embarcadero Road, Suite 200
Palo Alto, CA 94303-3318
(650) 354-0733
www.dalailamafoundation.org
The Dalai Lama is the world's foremost Buddhist leader. In the YouthMoves program, teenagers from all over the world explore and communicate about peace and ethics in our modern world.

Holiday's Yoga Center
510 S.W. Third Avenue, Suite 210
Portland, OR 97204
(503) 224-8611
www.holidaysyogacenter.com
One of the early pioneers to develop yoga programming just for teenagers, Holiday's has a great Web site. Check it out.

Yoga4Teens
YogaMinded
282 Monterey Drive
Laguna Beach, CA 92651
www.yogaminded.com
Amazing yogini Christy Brock works with teenagers all over the country. She teaches at the Omega Institute's teen summer camp, too. See the Web site to order her video *Yoga4Teens*.

YogaKids International
2501 Oriole Trail, Suite 66
Long Beach, IN 46360
(800) 968-0694
www.yogakids.com
Mostly for little kids, but the company also sponsors family yoga vacations to cool places.

Omega Institute for Holistic Studies
150 Lake Drive
Rhinebeck, NY 12572
(800) 944-1001
www.eomega.org
A two-week coed summer camp for teenagers includes yoga and other mind, body, and spirit programming in a beautiful rural setting.

Index

Index